2022

BIPOLAR….. MAYBE?

VOLUME TWO

John Barrett

Copyright © John Barrett

All rights reserved. No part of this publication may be reproduced, stored in a retrieval system, or transmitted in any form or by any means without the prior written permission of the publisher.

BIPOLAR.....MAYBE?
(Volume Two)

ACKNOWLEDGEMENTS

Jane Bloomfield, Lorraine Swift, Pauline Brown, Davey Barrett, Pat Barrett, David Barrett, Patsy Barrett, Ernie Barrett, Lee Barrett, David Brown, Helen Bell, Michael Barrett, Roy Cashman and Andrew Bloomfield

BIPOLAR…..MAYBE?
(Volume Two)

This, the second part of Bipolar…..Maybe?
continues to see if some of the things I've done in my
earlier life were a direct result of having bipolar before
I knew I had it, or even what it was.

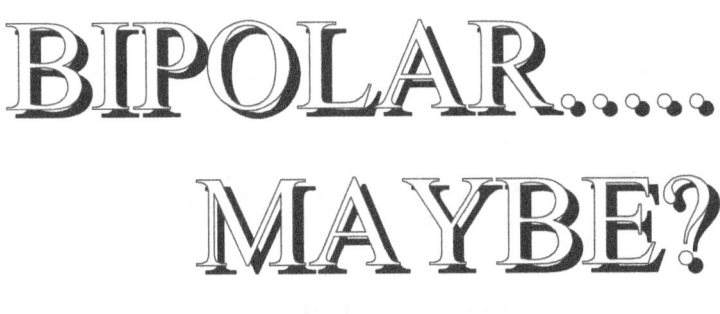

VOLUME TWO

As before, many of the names have been changed.

For
Patricia
or as she's more
commonly known,
Pat or mum

Front cover photo used with kind permission of David Barrett.

BIPOLAR…..MAYBE?
(Volume Two)

Also by the same author

**Frank Fireball in
Pronounced Dop-el-geng-er**

The Adventures of Dustman Dan

Bipolar..... Me?

Bipolar….. Maybe?
Volume One

Bipolar….. Definitely!

**Frank Fireball & the Confounding Case
of
Paxomus Maxomus**

A Saturday in Mid September

Writing under the name Sydney Novak

**An Empty Kettle
(parts 1 & 2)**

BIPOLAR…..MAYBE?
(Volume Two)

…the BBC mini-series from 1985 called Edge of Darkness, starring the late, great Bob Peck. Not only is the story by Troy Kennedy-Martin brilliant, along with the direction by Martin Campbell, it is made in such a way that doesn't insult the viewer's intelligence and has no need to rely on fancy editing or a pounding soundtrack. Instead, we have a programme given the time to tell its story at a leisurely pace, and the score by Michael Kamen and Eric Clapton is beautifully haunting and really adds to the tension of the piece. The acting from all concerned is excellent, with you truly believing in the characters on the screen. I won't tell you the story because it will spoil it, but I warn you, if you prefer the way dramas are made today, then I would suggest not bothering, you would probably be bored to tears. I honestly believe dramas such as Edge of Darkness wouldn't get made today; the viewing tastes of the general public has changed too much and that is very sad. Don't get me wrong, there are some fine dramas out there with great story lines, it's just that they don't have…. how can I put it? A certain something

The first time it was ever shown was on BBC2 on a Monday evening, when I was due to go down to the pub to meet up with my mates, which was usual every Monday night. It was pouring down outside and I really wasn't in the mood to go out, and so turned the TV on just as Edge of Darkness was about to start, figuring I'd watch it for about twenty minutes until the rain hopefully stopped. Needless to say, by the time twenty minutes had passed, I was completely hooked and wasn't going anywhere. Granted, I admit the first fifteen minutes are slow and I was about to give up on it, but everything suddenly changes from that point onwards and it really is a guessing game about who did what, from that moment on. So, for the next six Mondays, I didn't go down the pub, and instead watched one of the best television drama the world has ever seen (no exaggeration!)

Needless to say, I've got it on DVD and have since seen it about ten times, and no doubt I will see it at least ten more times in the future…. because I enjoy the finer things in life.

BIPOLAR…..MAYBE?
(Volume Two)

The views expressed in this book
are solely that of the author and if any one feels
uncomfortable or disagrees with them,
the afore mentioned author suggests they use the pages
within as karzy paper or perhaps as paper mache in order to
create an ornate vase or a hideous fire breathing dragon,
or a statue of the mother-in-law.
Hold on a minute, those last two examples are pretty much
the same thing…still I suppose it's like killing two birds with
one stone.
Yay!

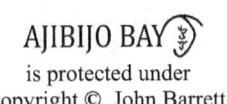

is protected under
copyright © John Barrett

BIPOLAR…..MAYBE?
(Volume Two)

Listed below are some more famous people who either have or had Bipolar Disorder
(the poor sods!)

Adam Ant (chapter 1) page: 13
Amy Winehouse (chapter 2) page: 27
Arthur Lipsett (chapter 3) page: 40
Axl Rose (chapter 4) page: 50
Ben Stiller (chapter 5) page: 60
Carrie Fisher (chapter 6) page: 70
Catherine Zeta-Jones (chapter 7) page: 84
Britney Spears (chapter 8) page: 98
Connie Francis (chapter 9) page: 108
Dusty Springfield (chapter 10) page: 114
Frank Bruno (chapter 11) page: 124
Gene Tierney (chapter 12) page: 132
Georg Cantor (chapter 13) page: 142
Gustav Mahler (chapter 14) page: 157
Jackson Pollock (chapter 15) page: 166
Jeremy Brett (chapter 16) page: 174
Mike Tyson (chapter 17) page: 181
Kurt Cobain (chapter 18) page: 188
Lily Allen (chapter 19) page: 194
Linda Hamilton (chapter 20) page: 201
Lou Reed (chapter 21) page: 213
Margot Kidder (chapter 22) page: 221
Naomi Sims (chapter 23) page: 228
Patricia Cornwell (chapter 24) page: 236
Patty Duke (chapter 25) page: 243
Marianne Joan Elliott-Said (chapter 26) page: 252
Paul Gascoigne (chapter 27) page: 260

BIPOLAR…..MAYBE?
(Volume Two)

Famous people continued

Rene Russo (chapter 28) page: 268
Jonathan Winters (chapter 29) page: 274
Robin Williams (chapter 30) page: 281
Sidney Sheldon (chapter 31) page: 287
Sinead O'Connor (chapter 32) page: 294
Stephen Fry (chapter 33) page: 301
Terry Hall (chapter 34) page: 312
Tom Waits (chapter 35) page: 320
Burgess Meredith (chapter 36) page: 325
Macy Gray (chapter 37) page: 332
Mariette Hartley (chapter 38) page: 341

BIPOLAR…..MAYBE?
(Volume Two)

PART ONE: TOIL
Page 11 - page 155

PART TWO: RELAXATION
Page 156 – page 234

PART THREE: RECREATION
Page 235 - page 318

PART FOUR:
WOULD THAT IT WERE
Page 319 – page 348

BIPOLAR…..MAYBE?
(Volume Two)

PART ONE: TOIL

PART ONE: TOIL

FORWARD:

Before we kick off proceedings, let's start with a short poem:

I like stalking Richard Dawkins
And his mate Chris Hitchens
If you ever lose your voice
You can always fit some kitchens

and perhaps a little song:

Oh, I do like to be rather rambunctious
Oh, I do like to be rather bum bee
With a rumpy pumpy pum
And a diddly did did dee
Rather rambunctious
Rather bum bee

There, that's better…... and now the story.

BIPOLAR…..MAYBE?
(Volume Two)

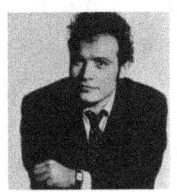

CHAPTER 1

Spring 2006

After working at my friend Simon's company for nine years, my heart just wasn't in it anymore and I quit in 2004 to try and continue my father-in-law's business of property developing. He had decided to retire the following year, and so along with his daughter (my wife Debbie) we thought it was worth giving it a go and I planned to help Gary (the main builder) in restoring run-down houses, before selling them for a profit. I had got to know Gary some years earlier when he worked on an extension for our first house and then a few years later, on our second home as well. On both occasions, I assisted him as much as I was able to, as did my father-in-law who is such a great bloke and basically, we were Gary's labourers, doing the fetching and carrying and any work that didn't entail having any particular skills. Debbie's dad warned us however that it was getting harder and harder to make a good living in the property game, which he put down to the ever-increasing number of people having the same idea, in the wake of all the TV shows being aired at the time. Even with that warning in mind however, we still decided to go ahead and things went quite well for the first two years, but eventually, my father-in-law's prediction proved accurate and things became a real struggle. The main problem we faced was buying properties for a cheap enough price in order to make a worthwhile profit, and it was at this point that my depression really started to kick in.

I mentioned in 'Volume One' about the spells of depression during my life before being diagnosed with bipolar, and how I thought everyone suffered with them, but this time was different and much more severe. I don't really know why it was so bad on this occasion (I'd been through plenty of hardships and difficult situations before) but bad it definitely was and I found myself going straight to bed as soon as I got home and not getting out of it until the following morning. I didn't have anything to eat and wouldn't talk to Debbie or see the kids, but instead went up to the bedroom as quickly as I could and pulled the duvet over my head (more often than not, without even bothering to get undressed) Debbie would come into the room and try to talk to me, but I wouldn't say anything and held my eyes as tightly shut as possible, trying to block her out. This went on for weeks and during the day, it was like I was on some kind of auto pilot, just going through the motions until I could get home and to bed again. It must have been so frustrating for Debbie because the same hardships that were happening to me were happening to her as well, and she just couldn't get a response out of me. Somehow, she eventually persuaded me to go see my doctor but when he diagnosed me as having depression, I did the typical thing and just thought I was feeling low and would snap out of it soon. The GP prescribed me some anti-depressants which I promised to take but as soon as I got home, I threw the prescription in the bin and lied to Debbie about my diagnosis.

Several weeks passed without any change in my condition and Debbie once again booked me an appointment with the GP, but this time she said she would go along with me. Needless to say, Debbie quickly discovered that I'd not been taking any meds, so the doctor prescribed them to me again and don't ask why, but this time I accepted I was suffering with depression and agreed to take the tablets. Being me though, a few days passed with there not being any change in my condition and I told Debbie the GP must have been wrong, but she pleaded with me to carry on with the meds and after a couple of weeks, I gradually started to notice a change in my condition. Finally, about a month later, I would describe my mood as fully returned to normal (whatever that is) and gradually as the weeks passed, I forgot not only about the depressive episode, but about ever having it in the first place. It's a strange thing that; it doesn't take long to forget how I was feeling until it comes back again (and come back it did)

Summer 1998
At the age of eight, my eldest son starting going to Judo lessons a couple of times a week after school and was really starting to enjoy it. After about three weeks of attending, his enthusiasm started to rub off on me and so I began to attend in the evenings with the same Sensei, but obviously in a class for adults, although I would have stood a better chance of being any good in

PART ONE: TOIL

the kid's class. One of the deciding factors in wanting to go, was working for my friend Simon's family company that made wooden pasting tables and step ladders, as the production manager. The business originated in Bethnal Green and had been there for many, many years but as housing developments grew around them, they became increasingly under pressure to relocate, which they eventually did, to Harlow in Essex. About six of their workforce were persuaded to carry on working for the company and a minibus was laid on, to transport them from London to Essex and back again in the evenings. I had previously worked for my own family's business which had unfortunately gone into liquidation during the recession in the early nineties, but I didn't have a clue when it came to making pasting tables and step ladders and so as a result, had a lot of learning to do. I reckon Simon's firm had forty odd (very odd!) people working on the shop floor and apart from the Bethnal Green guys and two older men from Harlow who'd had previous experience working with wood, the rest of the workforce was made up with school leavers. None of these kids had qualifications in anything (much like myself at their age) and didn't understand the concept of arriving on time (very unlike myself) and as it appeared to me, weren't willing to work either. As a result of this, they were all on a minimum wage, which was only right because most of them didn't give a shit, but now and again, you would get someone who seemed to have a bit of savvy. These people quickly improved not only in the quality of their work but also in the speed of it too, and the only major thing I disagreed with, was they should have been offered slightly more money which would have done two things: It would have made them want to stay with the business and secondly to encourage them to improve even further, but they stayed on the same minimum wage and as a result, became disgruntled with the whole place. The company must have had new people starting about three times a week and you could tell just by looking at most of them if they were going to last until the Friday or not. Simon's dad Fred would give each new comer a short interview and no matter how bad they were, he'd employ them and send 'em down to me.

I remember him showing one kid around the factory and I thought to myself, "I'll give him two hours tops, before he walks out"

I was well out on my calculations though, because when he started a quarter of an hour later (they were always accepted because of the cheap labour) I put him on the assembly line where the legs and metal stays were fitted into the pasting tables and he walked out after just ten minutes. Ah…the great British workforce…best in the world, but what else did I expect, because when one of them (or three) wouldn't turn up for work, I'd ring their home number only for it to be answered with, "Yeh?"

"Hello, is that the home of Bradley Jones?"

"Who wants to know?"

"I'm calling from Bradley's place of work" (I was guessing it was his father I was speaking to and why wasn't he at bloody work either? Probably signed off because of some fictitious bad back injury and claiming benefits)

"And?"

"He hasn't come into work this morning…is he unwell?"

"How should I fucking know! Hold on a minute" then the phone would go all muffled by someone placing their hand over the mouthpiece followed by, "BRAD! BRAD!....ARE YOU UP THERE?"

"YEH!"

"IT'S SOME BLOKE WANTS TO KNOW IF YOU'RE GOING INTO WORK TODAY!"

"I'VE GOT A BELLY ACHE!"

"WHAT….ANOTHER ONE?"

"YEH AND THIS ONE IS WORSE THAN BEFORE"

The line would then become clear again with, "No…he ain't going in!" and then the phone went dead. It was like that 90% of the time and I found it totally pointless ringing them up in the first place, but that was the policy of the company. If that's how their parents behaved, then it's no wonder they turned out the same way, but what has any of this got to do with Judo I hear you ask. At least once a week, a couple of the school leavers would end up fighting over something trivial and it was down to me to split them up, which I usually managed to do; not by steaming in and dragging them apart but rather by alleviating the situation and making light of it.

"Now, now children, we're all friends here," I would say and that would usually stop them for a moment before I continued with, "That's better…now give him a big cuddle or if you're not willing to do that, then at least shake hands"

Most of the time they would start to laugh at the cuddle bit but on the odd occasion, they'd take no notice and

BIPOLAR…..MAYBE?
(Volume Two)

that's when I'd have to step in. I'm not an aggressive person in any way whatsoever and therefore found it pretty difficult asserting myself in that kind of manner but once again, just by standing between the two individuals and slowly pushing them apart usually done the trick. Now and again however, one of them would turn aggressive towards me and I found it difficult trying to calm them down and it must have come across to the onlookers as a sign of weakness.

Fred would employ absolutely anyone, and on one occasion he hired this kid who must have been eighteen or nineteen in age and in stones, and came from a gypsy family. He was bloody hopeless, the useless lump and was always larking about, which meant I had to reprimand him time and time again. I was upstairs in the office one time and just before I was about to go down on the shop floor again, I stared out of the window in the showroom, which overlooked the entire length of the factory, and could see the gypsy kid feeding long lengths of timber into the machine that planed them down to the correct size, which was situated at the far end of the building. Nothing wrong with that because he was supposed to be doing it but he wasn't supposed to have a lighter held underneath the wood with the flame set on high. Blimey, I've just realised how much my eyesight has deteriorated since then because there's no way now I would be able to see that far. Of course the timber was moving too quickly for it to set alight but that wasn't the point and one of the main rules was 'no naked flames on the shop floor' "That's it," I said to myself, "I've given him so many chances but enough is enough," and then I made my

PART ONE: TOIL

way down the metal staircase and began to walk to the end of the factory. As I got closer and closer, I could see he was still doing it until he spotted me coming and put the lighter in his pocket.

"I've given you so many chances," I explained to him, "But this is the last…you're sacked"

"Sacked! What for?" he yelled.

"I saw you with the lighter, holding it under the timber"

"What lighter?"

"The one you put in your pocket when you saw me coming"

At the same time I was thinking to myself, "What am I doing this fucking shit for? If they hired someone half decent, then the job would get done much quicker and there wouldn't be any of this crap to deal with.

Okay…it would cost a bit more but at least the job would get done without any hold ups.

"You can't sack me!" he screamed

"Yes I can and I've just done it," I replied as I leant forward and turned the machine off.

"Hey…what's going on?" came the muffled voice of Bill at the other end of the machine. Bill was one of the Bethnal Green guys who originated from Jamaica and he drove the minibus too. His voice was muffled because he always wore a dust mask and the only times I didn't see him wearing one was either when he was eating his lunch or as he was leaving to go home.

"Sorry Bill mate," I replied, "Can you take over here and get someone to go on your end"

"Hmmm…. yeh… okay," he grumbled.

"Come on," I said to the gypsy kid (sorry, not very P.C but traveller just doesn't sound right) "Follow me"

BIPOLAR…..MAYBE?
(Volume Two)

"You fucking cunt!" he yelled so eloquently, but started to walk alongside me (well…wobble) as I made my way back up to the other end of the building. As he walked, he had his head down to the ground and said nothing, and then all of a sudden, he lunged towards me but luckily, I guessed he might do something like that and stepped out of the way. Another of the Bethnal Green crew was this guy called Leslie who had mild learning difficulties and was also extremely over weight, and I always got on really well with him. It sounds absolutely terrible now because I work with people with L.D but at that time, I (along with everybody else I knew) would have described him as 'a bit simple'

That wasn't meant in a derogatory way, it was the only description I knew and I'd certainly never heard the term 'learning difficulties' before. Anyway, Leslie appeared from nowhere, wrapped his arms around this kid and started to march him in the direction we'd been headed. Unbeknown to me, Simon and his brother Matthew were watching the scene unfold from the upstairs window in the showroom and as me, Leslie and the gypsy kid reached the bottom of the metal staircase (which was right next to the exit) they opened the showroom door and started to walk down the stairs. The kid was effing and blinding at me when Simon said, "I think it's time you left"

Just as he was about to walk to the exit, he turned around and spat straight in my face, and it was at that point I just lost it and threw him down to the ground.

"Mother fucker!" I yelled as Matthew pulled me away from him and when he got back on his feet, he made his

PART ONE: TOIL

way to the exit whilst yelling, "You haven't heard the last of this!"

I'll be honest with you…all this writing about having fights etc bores me to death and I'll admit myself, it's a pretty naff start to the book but it is relevant to the Judo lessons. Maybe I shouldn't have mentioned the Judo lessons in the first place but they too are relevant to the incidents at Simon's place. Hold on a minute…if I didn't write about the Judo, then I wouldn't have to write about the factory fights and then…. oh, I don't know, it's all a vicious circle (or if you don't like fighting like me) a pacifist's circle. I've got to write about something ain't I or else there'd be no bleedin' book.

Back to the boring bit. Just before it was time to go at five in the afternoon, Simon said I should check my rear-view mirror as I drove home because gypsies are as tough as nails and can hold a grudge for a long time. He didn't have to tell me that because I knew it for myself already but luckily, no one followed me and I didn't hear anything else afterwards. So that was one of the reasons I thought it would be a good idea to learn Judo, in order to protect myself, but the other reason was I figured it was a good way to keep fit at the same time. Simon knew I didn't do all that macho bullshit and to me, he was always someone who felt like they had to prove themselves. Me and our other mate Robert were totally opposite to that and when we all used to go out, me and Rob just wanted to have a laugh and mess about, whereas Simon and Ed (another friend) put on the hard man act. Life is way too short for all that crap, give me a joke and a good sense of humour any day of the week. Me, Simon and Ed would usually go for a drink every Friday evening (by this time, Rob had emigrated to Marbella with his twin sister Julie to be near their mum and dad) and our other mates, Chris and Jerrod had moved near to the Chelmsford area which was about twenty miles away.

This would have been just before Barrett's went into liquidation and for over a year, I kept all of the hard times I was going through, away from Simon and Ed. We were going out to have a good time and I didn't want to bring the mood down but even so, the both of them were always so serious. I remember on one Friday evening, we were drinking in the Railway Arms in Theydon and Simon asked me, "Where do you see yourself in a year's time?"

"Hmmm…a year's time eh?" I replied while rubbing my chin and then took three steps to the side to move slightly along the bar before continuing with, "Just about here"

Simon gave an unconvincing smile and said, "And what about a year after that?"

I moved back to my original position and said, "Right here!"

Neither Simon or Ed seemed to find it very amusing and I thought to myself, "You pair of miserable old gits!" and longed so much for Rob to be back in the country.

So, telling Simon I was starting Judo lessons made him think I was finally going to become like him, but I knew that even in the unlikely event I'd become a black belt, I would always be that crazy Johnny Boy, who messing about was a main thing when it came to living my life.

PART ONE: TOIL

Matthew had done Judo for a while and why oh why did I open my big mouth and tell him I was having lessons? One evening after work, it was just me and Matthew left upstairs and I was due to go to a lesson. When we locked up and were about to get in our cars, I opened my boot and put the clothes I'd changed from into it and then slammed it shut.
"Fuck it!" I said.
"What's the matter?" asked Matthew.
"My car keys are in the boot and it's locked along with all the doors.
"Have you got a spare?"
"Yeh…at home"
"Ah!"
So I rang my wife Debbie and she had to drive the half hour journey to bring me the spare keys. Fair play to Matthew because he waited with me, but the worst thing I could have told him was that I would miss my lesson. I just assumed that Simon had told him about the Judo but he obviously hadn't because Matthew suggested we do some moves and I felt like a right fucking idiot as people walked past staring at us. He grabbed the collar of my tee shirt and said, "Get out of that," which I did and then I had to do the same thing to him. Matthew must be six foot five and is really slim and clearly thought very highly of himself, to say the least.

"And of course, your balance improves significantly when you have mastered the technique!" he enthusiastically explained.

I had to admit I agreed with him because I'd noticed the difference in myself but just to prove his point, he lifted his elongated left leg and pointed it straight out, vertically in front of him.

"I am able to stay in this position for several minutes!" he enthused before his left foot pointed forward also, in my direction.

"Yeh...really good," I said while thinking to myself, "Come on Debbie... hurry up for fucks sake!"

"And when you are finally able to reach this standard," he continued whilst balanced on his right leg, "you will then be able to do this!"

Somehow...don't ask me how because I don't particularly know or care, he started to swivel round on his right foot while keeping his stretched left leg stuck out in front of him. He then pointed the foot at a clump of trees at the end of the street whilst placing both his hands on his hips. Just at that moment, Debbie pulled up next to us.

"Thank fuck for that!" I whispered under my breath.

"What was that?" asked Matthew.

"I said, thanks for waiting with me"

The first few Judo lessons didn't involve Judo at all but was rather about exercising, be it running up and down the length of the hall where the lessons were being held or doing star jumps or press ups or whatever. Before starting, I thought those exercises were going to kill me because I hadn't been keeping fit, but they weren't too bad at all and I realised that the amount of rushing around I did at work, was keeping me in good shape without realising it. It was only on the third lesson that we started performing some Judo moves, but they were solo efforts and not against an opponent. I was really enjoying it and it got to the stage where I couldn't wait to finish work and get there as quickly as possible. It wasn't until week five that we were teamed up with a partner and had to use the moves we'd learned against each other but without any actual physical contact.

"Fine," I thought, "I'm still really enjoying this. I'll be the next Bruce Lee before I even know it!"

The same thing happened the following lesson and it was only when week seven arrived, that we had to attempt to hit our partner and they had to try and block the moves. My partner's name was also John and it was his turn first to try and hit me and I successfully blocked each of his moves.

"Watch out Chuck Norris!" I told myself but then it was my turn to hit John.

I couldn't do it.

Even though I knew he was going to block my moves, I just couldn't get myself to try and hit him.

"Come on John…what are you waiting for?" he asked with a confused expression on his face.

"I can't do it John," I replied.

"Why not?"

"I don't know but I just can't," and that's when I realised Judo just wasn't for me.

To hit somebody when they have done nothing bad towards me is just not in my makeup and that was the last lesson I ever did. I know it's a sport and shouldn't be looked at as if it were a fight caused by a genuine argument or whatever but that's not how I was made and I'd much rather be like how I am naturally….just John who likes to see the funny things in life and not take it too seriously.

CHAPTER 2

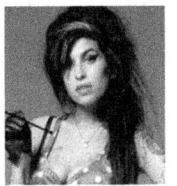

There were two lorry drivers at Simon's place, the first being Bob who drove a unit that pulled a forty-foot and a thirty-foot trailer, which the company owned and the second driver was a guy called Ricky who drove the box van. Bob lived in the unit permanently and because he liked a drink, it could be a nightmare trying to wake him up on a Monday morning when he was supposed to be going on his deliveries. He'd fitted curtains to the inside of the unit and they would be pulled shut as I stood by the driver's door, asking him if he was awake while looking down at my feet, only to see I was standing in a puddle of sick.
"Bob?" I'd call out, "Are you up yet?"
Silence…and so I knocked gently on the door.
"Bob!"
"Fuck off!" he'd growl in a gravelly voice which was mainly caused by the 120 cigarettes he smoked every day (no exaggeration)
Next to where he parked the unit was a dustbin which would regularly be filled to the brim with empty fag packets.
"Bob…you should have left three hours ago"
"Fuck off!"

PART ONE: TOIL

I'd then go and have to explain to Fred that he wouldn't budge. If it had been anybody else, Fred would have gone mad but Bob was a one off who'd drive all over the country, from down in Cornwall all the way up to Scotland. Okay, a lot of lorry drivers do that, but the trailer he'd be pulling was usually filled completely up with paste tables and ladders that were all loaded by hand. It would take five of us, most of the day to fill it up with the pasting tables stood on their sides along the width of the trailer, four tiers high with ladders on top of that. Bob would have to unload it by hand, all by himself and there could be as many as thirty different delivery points (usually to shops situated in a high street) Fred wasn't stupid and knew he'd never get another person like Bob and would therefore ring up the customers and explain that their deliveries would be several hours late.

With Ricky however it was a totally different story because Fred could easily get another driver for the box van at any time and he would get in as many deliveries as possible during the course of the day. Ricky must have been in his mid-fifties, was about five foot two, had jet black hair that he'd obviously dyed and it was combed in the style of a teddy boy from a bygone era, complete with a quiff at the front. On one occasion, I was talking to John who worked upstairs in the office at five to five in the afternoon. Ricky had been out for most of the day doing deliveries in the box van, when he pulled up outside and came upstairs.

"I'm really sorry John," he said, "but I ran out of time to get the last drop off done"

"What time did they shut then?" I asked.

BIPOLAR.....MAYBE?
(Volume Two)

"They were doing a stock take and wouldn't take any more deliveries after four o'clock...do you think you should let Fred know?" he replied with a look of absolute terror on his face.

"Yeh...I suppose I'd better," I replied before picking up the phone on John's desk and dialling through to Fred's office.

"Yes John?" came the voice on the other end of the line.

"This is the other John...I'm calling from John's desk," I explained.

"Yes John...how can I help you?"

"Ricky has just got back and says he didn't have time to do the last drop"

The line went quiet for a moment and I gazed over at Ricky who was staring at me with an equal mixture of concern and fear.

"Hello Fred?"

"Tell him he's a fucking useless cunt!"

He shouted so loud I was convinced Ricky must have heard, so I gave him a reassuring smile and he smiled back at me.

"Go on!" yelled Fred, "Tell him he's a cunt!"

"Yeh...I will in a minute," I replied and with that, Fred hung up.

"He's not angry with me is he?" asked Ricky.

"Well...let's just say you're not in his good books at the moment"

"Oh dear"

Just then in the distance, was the sound of Fred's office door being forcibly opened, followed by loud footsteps walking through the showroom.

"I'd get off pretty sharpish if I was you," said John sat

behind his desk and with that, Ricky turned on his Cuban heels and rushed over to the main office door. He'd just about managed to get halfway outside when Fred walked in and yelled, "Ricky! Get back in here now!"

"I'm sorry Fred bu... bu... but they wouldn't let me unload," stuttered Ricky.

"What are you fucking talking about... wouldn't let you?"

"They were doing a stock...."

"John... get them on the phone right now!" shouted Fred, cutting Ricky off short.

"There'll probably be no answer, it's gone five," said John.

"Give me the number and I'll ring them myself!" said Fred as he walked over to the dispatch desk and sat behind it.

"Well... I'll be going now," said Ricky in a meek voice as he opened the door again, "It's gone five o'clock"

"Get back in here now!" yelled Fred and with that, Ricky shuffled back into the office while staring down at the ground.

"Ah yes... hello there," said Fred into the phone in a quiet and polite manner, "Our driver was supposed to drop off your paste tables this afternoon but failed to make the delivery"

"It wasn't that Fred, it was...."

"I understand that," said Fred into the phone, "but we were told the delivery was urgent and had to be with you today"

That was a total lie but Fred was determined to get that delivery out.

BIPOLAR…..MAYBE?
(Volume Two)

"I see… I see… so what time do you open in the morning?"

Ricky looked over to me and John and knew what was coming.

"Seven o'clock… yes, that's absolutely fine. He'll be waiting outside when you arrive in the morning. Thank you and goodbye.

"Right! You fucking heard that!" yelled Fred after hanging up the phone, "You need to be here by six so you can make the delivery in time!"

"Yes Fred but…"

"And don't let me down again!"

"No Fred" he replied and with that he trundled off home with his tail firmly between his legs.

Ricky saw himself as a budding artist and from time to time he'd bring in some of his watercolours to show us. A few of them weren't bad but there was one of his wife in the nude that looked like she was a fucking gorilla and all of us struggled not to burst out laughing. She was standing up but hunched over with her arms dangling by her sides and her black pubic hair seemed to rise all the way up to her belly button.

"What do you think?" he asked me.

"Yeh… really good Ricky, what is it?" I asked.

"That's my wife!" he replied with a look of satisfaction on his face, "I'm particularly proud of this one!"

"She's a real stunner," I said and quickly walked into the tea room for a cigarette before I started laughing in front of him.

Ricky followed me in and said, "If you want me to do a painting of your wife, just let me know"

PART ONE: TOIL

"What? Er... yeh... thanks mate, I'll let her know," I replied and had a vision of Debbie standing buck naked in the middle of Ricky's living room as he transformed her into some kind of hideously hairy abomination! (I was gonna write, no change there then as a joke but thought better of it... hold on, I've just written it... whoops)

About ten years before I started at Simon's company, several Polish businesses approached his firm about supplying their own pasting tables and although the profit margin wasn't that great, they agreed. Being in Poland, these companies could source their timber locally, whereas Simon's firm had to buy it in from Sweden, and three of the Polish firms delivered the pasting tables using their own transport. We would usually stack two lines of tables on a pallet, twenty-five high so it made a pallet of fifty, but on the Polish lorries, a further ten either side were strapped separately to make it a pallet of seventy. The main problem with these deliveries was that the pasting tables would move about even though they had four separate straps going around the whole pallet. We would end up having to unload most of it by hand and put the damaged ones to one side, which could be as many as three hundred on a particularly bad day. It was such a time consuming job and if none of the pasting tables had shifted, then it would have been an absolute doddle unloading the whole thing by forklift. On one occasion it was tea break and I was upstairs talking to John when I saw one of these Polish lorries pull up outside.
"Here we go again," I mumbled to John and just as I

was about to walk away from the window, I noticed the canvas top of the trailer lift slightly to a point, before it split and a knife blade came through. The knife cut a three-foot line in the material and then a man's head popped through.

"Here John, look at this," I said.

The man pulled himself out of the trailer and then leant back down to pull three of his friends out too.

"I don't fucking believe it!" said John as they climbed down the side of the trailer before running to the end of the street into a small wooded area.

What surprised me the most was the fact there was only about a twelve-inch space between the top of the pasting tables and the roof of the trailer. They must have been laid down flat all the way from the docks on the other side of the water and it made me realise just how desperate some of these people are to get into England. We used to do overtime on a Saturday morning (although I didn't get paid for it because it was expected of me) and on one of these mornings on a cold winter's day, I pulled up outside the building to be faced with four Polish lorries all lined up in a row. It was freezing cold, the sky was grey and pissing down, and the strong wind was almost blowing the rain vertically.

"Triffick!" I said to myself as I got out the car and just knew that each of the lorries' paste tables would be all over the place owing to the ferry crossing in high winds and I was absolutely right.

Somehow, we managed to get all four of them unloaded by twelve and in total there must have been over a thousand damaged paste tables. We had three forklifts, one diesel and the other two electric, plus one side-loader which could carry long lengths of timber. Seeing as I'd come from my own family business and used to go there on my school holidays, I had been driving forklifts from about the age of twelve and I'm not trying to blow my own trumpet, but I was very good at it too. Bob the lorry driver would always try and wind me up because I'm normally (not high or low, with the old you know what) a very laid-back person and I would always tell him he was wasting his breath because, "I am immune"

"Ain't you done that bit of a job yet?" he'd bark with a grin on his face and a cigarette stuck out the corner of his mouth while I'd be loading up his trailer.

I suppose he was about fifty at the time and had long hair pulled into a pony tail and a beard as long as Dusty Hill's and Billy Gibbons' out of ZZ Top. As well as delivering pasting tables and step ladders to high street decorating shops that all had to be unloaded by hand, Bob would also deliver to larger companies that had forklifts and therefore the goods would be loaded onto pallets. For 95% of the time, Bob would either take the piss out of me or try and wind me up, but on that rare 5% he would say, "You're the best forklift driver I have ever seen"

Bearing in mind he would deliver to companies all over the entire country, that is quite a complement. Cheers Bob, you miserable git. I'm joking because that was all an act he put on and I was genuinely really fond of him. There were two other Polish companies that delivered to us but their loads came in on forty-foot containers that had to be collected from Tilbury Docks. This job

BIPOLAR…..MAYBE?
(Volume Two)

fell down to the Hogger twins from Bethnal Green who I'm guessing were in their mid-sixties. They were a right couple of characters who would supply me with beer and cigarettes and bottles of wine for Debbie, from a connection they had at the docks. Their unit and flatbed trailer were on their last legs (or should I say wheels?) and were always breaking down. On one occasion after dropping off a container to us, they were driving back home along Lee Bridge Road in Leyton, which is a very busy road and is always teaming with pedestrians, when Georgie (who was driving) looked out of his window to see a wheel rolling along the road and overtaking him.

"Look at that Bobbie," he said to his brother, "some silly cunt has lost their wheel!" and with that, they both burst out laughing.

Suddenly a car pulled up alongside them and the bloke driving started beeping his horn and pointing at the back of their unit.

"What's up with him?" said Bobbie.

"Dunno?" replied Georgie while winding down his window.

"What's the matter mate?" he called out to the driver.

"One of your wheels has come off!"

"Eh?"

"I said, one of your wheels has just come off!"

With that, Georgie looked at the wheel speeding off ahead of him as it mounted the pavement and struck an old man who hadn't managed to get out of the way in time. Because the unit had a double wheel base at the rear, Georgie hadn't noticed when one of them came off, but he did notice as it knocked over the old man

PART ONE: TOIL

like a bowling pin and who was now lying face down as everybody else on the pavement ran out of the wheel's path. Each of the wheels must have been four foot high and even with three people; it would have still been a struggle to pick one up.

"Aw my gawd!" said Bobbie, "What are we gonna do?"

"Just keep going and pretend we didn't notice," replied his brother.

Just then, both of them noticed a police car coming down the road in the opposite direction and it was bound to stop when it saw the old man lying on the pavement.

"We're gonna have to pull over," said Georgie, "otherwise they'll do us for fleeing the scene of the accident"

So that's what they did and luckily for them the old man wasn't seriously injured (which was a miracle) and he didn't want to sue, but they still had to go to court to decide the fine they should be given.

"How did it go?" I asked Georgie the following day when they dropped off a container.

"They fined us five hundred quid!"

"Shit…that's a bummer!" I replied

"The old boy the wheel knocked over was there too," said Bobbie.

"How did you know it was him?" I asked, "You never saw his face when he was on the pavement"

"Because he had a great big tyre mark running up his back," replied Georgie and with that, both of them burst out laughing.

Unloading the containers in the summer was a nightmare because they were like ovens inside and I

BIPOLAR.....MAYBE?
(Volume Two)

remembered reading in the paper one time about fifty illegal immigrants dying in the heat as they attempted to smuggle themselves into the U.K. It must have been an awful way to go and I seem to remember the only survivor was a two-year-old girl who was saved just in time. The containers could hold twenty-eight pallets of fifty paste tables, with a further fourteen packed loosely on top and you had to use a step ladder to get to them. When I would help to unload them and climb up the ladder, my bald bonce would sometimes touch the roof of the container which was red hot in the summer sun. Man that bloody hurt! By far the majority of paste tables sold to our customers had hardboard surfaces and increasingly, our own workforce made plywood tables and heavy-duty ones. Once brought into the factory, the pallets of fifty hardboard tables would be stacked two high and in five lines of sixty pallets, and when driving a forklift down an empty line with two full lines either side, it reminded me of Star Wars when Luke Skywalker is flying his X-Wing along the trench of the Death Star near the end of the film. The forklift only had two inches of clearance on either side and I'd have to drive at full speed most of the time because we were running tight on time (as usual)

One of the electric forklifts had the forks removed and replaced with these two flat metal plates which stood vertically and were covered in a thick rubber sheet on the inside. The plates were four foot square and would open up or close together to grab hold of the pallets and that came in handy when some of the Polish pallets were all over the place because the metal plates could sometimes straighten them up. We had two shrink wrapping machines which had carousels the pallets would be placed on, and after tying the shrink wrap to one of the blocks on the pallets; it would slowly start to rise up to the top of the paste tables and back down again as the carousel turned round. Well, that was the fully automatic one but the other had to be operated by hand which meant having a permanently sticky hand where the shrink wrap was pulled tight by the palm of your hand. By far our biggest customer was B&Q who could have up to as many as ten loads a week and even more at Easter time because that's when a lot of people do some decorating (apparently) We also supplied Homebase, Wickes, Do It All (which later became Focus) and Great Mills, as well as some others who I can't remember because my mind has gone completely blank.

The pallets that the Polish paste tables came in on, were exactly the same size as two stacks of tables side by side and as a result, twenty-eight pallet loads would fit onto a forty-foot trailer. Homebase however, had their pasting tables loaded onto blue CHEP pallets which were 1200 x 800mm in dimension and were bigger than the Polish pallets. This being the case, only twenty-six would fit onto a forty-foot trailer but increasingly, each of these companies renewed their old trailers to new forty-five-foot ones that could hold twenty-eight pallet loads of paste tables (confused yet?)

We called the CHEP pallets blue and the unstained ones of the same size were known as white. Whereas Homebase would deliver the blue pallets back to us, B&Q kept the white ones and so we had to buy more to replenish our stocks. B&Q had so much purchasing power that when they were planning to open a new store (at the time they had over 200) anywhere in the country, they would cover their costs by charging their suppliers. They justified this by telling the suppliers that each new store they opened would mean more business for the likes of us, but in reality, it was daylight robbery. We had to wait three months to receive a cheque from these big companies, but they would receive payment from their customers immediately when they purchased something in one of their stores. Hmm… it just doesn't seem fair to me, but that's business for you.

PART ONE: TOIL

CHAPTER 3

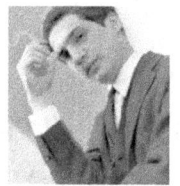

Autumn 2000
The outside loading yard at Simon's place was on a slope which ran downwards to a large set of wooden gates, and the main set of shutters to the factory were half way up the length of the building. The company had recently purchased another business in Haverhill which was about a forty minute drive away and made wooden bathroom cabinets and mirrors. Simon spent most of the week driving up there, which meant I was left solely in charge of running things down on the shop floor. I can remember vividly after three weeks of being on my own, my confidence starting to lift to another level and I was like someone on speed, rushing all over the place. In all the time I had been at Simon's firm, I hadn't been what I'd describe as my normal self but now I was the one making most of the decisions, my self-esteem returned in a massive way and it's only looking back now that I realise, I was experiencing a bipolar high, albeit it in a semi-controlled way.

After eight months of running things on my own downstairs, Fred came up to me one Friday afternoon and said, "We've been trying to reach the three-million-pound turnover mark for a long time and have just succeeded in doing so. That was achieved in no small part due to you... very well done"

"Thanks Fred," I replied but knew the only way that had happened was because I was willing to work alongside the rest of the workforce.

It was totally different to how Simon would have done things and I'm not saying my way was right or wrong, it's just the way I did things and I think I got much more respect from the guys because they could see I was willing to muck in.

So Simon was running the place up in Haverhill with a skeleton crew of some of their old workforce and they were basically assembling bathroom cabinets with parts they still had in stock. Once they neared the end of this stock, a decision had to be made whether they ordered in more materials or to take some of our paste table components up there and get the small workforce to assemble them. They decided on the latter, which meant Bob had to drive there with a trailer full of rims and pallets of hardboard etc, a couple of times a week. I mentioned earlier that we had a forty-foot trailer and a thirty-foot one and while Bob was out delivering with the forty-footer, I was loading up the shorter one with the forklift. One of the guys called Kevin (he was one of the better workers) and James (another forklift driver) were on the thirty-foot trailer with a pump-up truck, ready for me to load them some pallets of stock. How a trailer works is like this: They usually have two or three rows of double wheels at the back end and a set of metal legs with small metal wheels up the other end. These legs are set about eight feet in from the very front

PART ONE: TOIL

of the trailer, so the unit has enough room to reverse onto it, and are adjustable so the driver can wind them up and down with a large metal handle situated at the top of the legs. When the trailer is standing on its own without the driver's unit attached, the legs are wound down just enough for the unit to be backed onto the front of the trailer and after hooking up the air brake connectors and electrical leads etc, the driver then winds the legs upwards so they are about twelve inches off the ground. The difference with our thirty-foot trailer however was that there were only a single set of wheels at the back, which equated to much less weight. Seeing as I wanted to get as much stuff loaded onto it as possible, I double stacked two pallets of hardboard on top of each other and loaded them first. Each pallet of hardboard had five hundred sheets on it and probably weighed one ton, so that meant Kevin and James had to struggle with the pump-up truck and pull along two tons of weight to the front of the trailer.
"I might as well do the same again," I told myself and lifted another double stack onto the back of the trailer with the forklift.
As I drove back into the factory, I decided to load up several pallets of rims next and after picking them up, I made my way back to entrance to the loading area.
EEEEEAAAAARRRRRRCCCCRRHHHHH!!!!!!!
"What the fuck is that noise?" I asked myself and then it was followed by a loud crashing sound.
"Fucking hell!" I said out loud as I drove outside and was confronted with the back of the trailer sticking eighteen feet up in the air. Stupidly, I had loaded the heaviest stuff first and should have never double

BIPOLAR…..MAYBE?
(Volume Two)

stacked the hardboard because as Kevin and James pulled the second lot to the front of the trailer and beyond the point where the legs were touching the ground, it caused the whole fucking thing to tip forward. Several deciding factors made it tip up, with the main one being far too much weight at the front of the trailer. It didn't help either that the loading area sloped downwards and the thirty foot trailer only had one set of double wheels at the back, so obviously the weight of the hardboard was greater that the weight of the trailer. I say obviously, well… it was obvious in hindsight but at the time it just didn't enter my head. I climbed down off the forklift and stared up at the opening of the trailer, high above my head.

"Kevin…. James…. are you okay?" I called out.

Total silence.

"Shit, I've killed them!" I thought to myself.

"Kev…. James?"

"Yeh," came a faint voice from high up in the air and then two sets of hands appeared at the back of the trailer before they pulled themselves upwards. Both their heads peered down at me and Kevin had a cut on his forehead with blood trickling down to just above his left eye.

"Are you both okay?" I asked and felt absolutely terrible for what I'd done.

"Yeh," they both mumbled and I couldn't figure out how they had managed to climb up the smooth surface of the trailer because it must have been at least at a thirty degree angle.

"Stay there," I called out to them (not that they were going anywhere) and got back on the forklift and

PART ONE: TOIL

picked up an empty blue pallet. After lifting the pallet up to them, they just about managed to climb onto it before I lowered them back down to the ground. Fortunately the cut on Kevin's head wasn't that bad and James didn't appear to have any injuries at all. Luckily (very luckily) for me, they had turned the double stack of hardboard around on the pump-up truck and were pushing it to the front of the trailer when it tipped up. If they had still been pulling the pallets when it tipped, then the full two tons would have crushed them and I would have killed them for sure. The pallets of hardboard were so heavy that the one they'd been pushing, slammed into the front end of the trailer and caused it to crack on the outside surface. At this time, Simon and Matthew's mum was bedridden at home with cancer and Fred was with her while Simon was at Haverhill. That left Matthew who was upstairs and I had to go and tell him what happened.
"Hi Matt," I called out as I walked into his office.
"Hello"
"Erm… I've had a slight accident with the trailer while loading it"
"What do you mean…. what's happened?" he asked.
"It's easier if you come and see for yourself," I replied and so he followed me downstairs.
"Ah… I've never seen that happen before," he said in a calm manner and I was really surprised because I thought he was going to be angry (he had a really bad temper on him)
After explaining what had happened, he shook his head as if to say, "I understand," and I went and got the side-loader because it was heavier than the forklifts, and

placed its forks under the front end of the trailer which was touching the ground. Even the big side-loader struggled to lift the trailer up straight again but it just about managed it and then I had to get a team of people to re-stack the hardboard onto new pallets and then take them off with the forklift before reloading it with the weight distributed evenly. I felt like such an idiot because I'd never done anything even remotely close to that before but Matthew just said, "Accidents happen, don't worry about it. The main thing is, no one was seriously injured"

I thought I was doing the right thing by loading as much hardboard onto the trailer as I could and the excessive weight just didn't occur to me. I should have loaded the hardboard last and not double stacked the pallets but one thing was for sure, it was a lesson learned the hard way and I knew it would never happen again.

When I eventually got home that night, I was in the shower when suddenly the vision of the tipped-up trailer came into my head and I began to burst out laughing. It's weird because I didn't find it funny but all I could see was Kevin and James' heads peering out over the end of the trailer and the more I thought about it, the more I started to laugh. I couldn't stop and at the same time, I kept saying over and over again, "I could have killed them! I could have killed them!"

I was laughing hysterically but like I said, I didn't find it amusing so maybe it was nervous laughter or the relief that they had both been okay… or it could even have been the bipolar I didn't know I had yet. Even now, over twenty years later, the thought of it makes me feel uneasy, but at least I don't laugh anymore.

PART ONE: TOIL

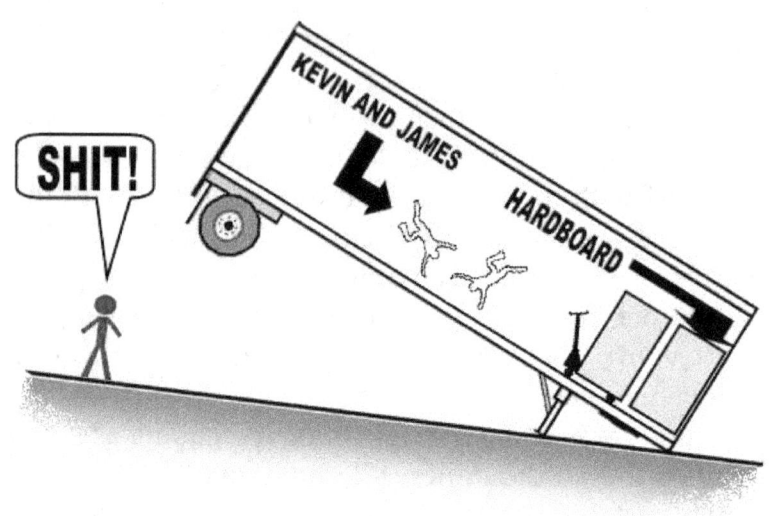

When Simon's mum was well, she would come to work on most days and although quietly spoken, she certainly didn't take any nonsense. Her and Fred's office was at the far end of the main offices which must have been over fifty feet away and with several closed doors in-between and yet you could hear Fred, Matthew and Simon having a heated discussion on numerous occasions. This would go on for several minutes before their loud voices were interrupted with, "Freddy... Matty... Simon... be quiet, all of you!" and nine times out of ten, total silence followed.

When she became ill, she didn't come into work as often and being quite a heavy-set woman (but by no means fat), it was awful to see her looking so skinny where the cancer had started to take its toll on her body, on the odd occasions she did come into work. She was a really well-spoken lady who had obviously been well educated and I always remember the time I lost my temper with the gypsy kid and she came up to me the next day and said, "I've heard you've been a naughty boy," with a smile on her face.

She was one of those people that got instant respect from those who met her, even for the first time (myself included) and I felt exactly the same way about Fred too. He'd spend more and more time looking after her before coming into work and the day before she died, Fred walked into the factory looking absolutely awful. His skin had turned grey and although he was naturally slim, he appeared to be skinny and I was worried he was going to collapse but somehow, he managed to stay on his feet and get through the day.

It soon became clear to me that the business in Haverhill was losing money hand over fist and so all the stock they had there, slowly came back to Harlow and began filling the place up. Once the Haverhill factory was cleared of everything (including office furniture and machinery) Simon's firm was forced to let the small skeleton crew go and the place was eventually shut down. The Harlow factory was becoming really tight for space and the six or seven office desks from Haverhill were stored in one of the old trailers we had outside. Unfortunately, this trailer had quite a few leaks and as a result, when it rained heavy, the inside of the trailer became increasingly damp and this caused the top of the desks to warp.

Fred being Fred, he put an ad in the local paper

PART ONE: TOIL

advertising the desks for sale (the only place they were fit for was the rubbish tip) and so we took them out of the trailer and put them in the warehouse. A few days later, a bloke turned up to take a look at them and I happened to be walking round the factory with Fred at the time. This would have been shortly after Simon's mum died but Fred was still able to put his salesman routine on as he was showing the guy these desks. Trying the drawers to see if they locked and opened and shut properly, the man took several steps back, crouched down on one knee and closed an eye. After several seconds, he stood up, turned to face Fred and said, "They're no good… all the tops are warped"

It was almost as if Fred never heard what he said and commented on the working order of the drawers.

"If you take all the desks, I'll throw in a couple of office chairs as well," he explained but failed to mention that the hydraulics on the chairs were playing up.

"What use are these desks to me?" replied the man, "The tops bow down in the middle"

I looked at Fred quickly and could tell he was thinking of something to say and I quickly answered, "That stops your pens from rolling off the edges"

Although my comment guaranteed no sale, Fred burst out laughing and it was great to see because he had been so depressed owing to his wife's death.

"Sorry Fred, I just couldn't resist it" I said once the man had gone, and was really surprised when he patted me on the back before walking up the metal staircase at the end of the warehouse and back to his office.

As more and more factory floor space filled up with paste tables, step ladders and bathroom cabinets, Fred told me to put the desks back in the leaking trailer and I had to laugh to myself because it was obvious they were never going to get sold.

Many of the bathroom cabinets were laminated and made from MDF, and most of the white ones had some of the laminate chipped off of them. Now bear in mind that these cabinets were to be sold to the likes of B&Q and Homebase, and Fred's unique method of repairing them. Any cabinets with obvious signs of damage were simply covered over with Tipp-ex to make them as good-as-new (not) and there was me, thinking I was a bodger.

Good old Fred.

PART ONE: TOIL

CHAPTER 4

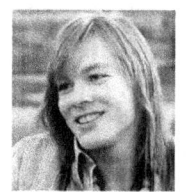

The Hoggers turned up with another container one Monday afternoon and as usual, they were having trouble with their unit, which they unhitched from the trailer. It appeared to be a problem with the battery because they couldn't get it to turn over, let alone start and so they rolled the unit down the slope of the outside loading area and stopped just by the worker's tea room which sat beneath Fred's office on the first floor. Bobbie was prodding around with a screwdriver while Georgie sat in the cabin with his feet up on the dashboard reading a paper, when suddenly, the screwdriver Bobbie was holding must have touched both battery terminals at once, causing it to explode. Simon happened to be in Fred's office at the time and as soon as he heard the bang, he looked out of the window and saw bits of battery flying up into the air (although at the time, he didn't know what it was)
Bobbie had his head only inches away from the battery when it blew up, so imagine the force of all those bits of plastic and acid hitting his face, especially considering that Simon saw bits flying past the window which was twelve feet up in the air. I happened to be in the tea room by the main office at the time, when

BIPOLAR.....MAYBE?
(Volume Two)

Georgie came in with Bobbie, who was holding his face in his hands. Georgie sat him down in a chair and then ran a tea towel under the cold water tap before handing it to Bobbie, who put it over his face. After Georgie had explained to me what had happened I said, "I'll make him a cup of tea"

"Yes...good idea," replied Georgie as I put the kettle on.

By this time, Simon walked into the tea room and asked Bobbie to remove the towel so he could look at his face. By some miracle the only obvious signs of injury were a few minor cuts and a couple of burns caused by the acid and luckily, his eyes didn't appear to be affected at all which was probably due to the fact he'd been wearing glasses. After making the cup of tea, I placed it down on the table in front of Bobbie but Georgie picked it up and took a big mouthful.

"Thanks John," he said, "I needed that to settle my nerves, I've come over all queer like!"

"That tea was meant for Bobbie," I explained.

"Oh was it? Sorry about that...you better make him another one"

Bobbie was whining in pain with the tea towel held firmly against his face again and Simon said, "It's really not that bad"

"Innit?" said Bobbie and removed the tea towel again as I handed him his cup of tea.

His mood changed considerably as he gulped down the tea and Georgie went out into the office to talk to Jackie about letting him know the serial number of the next container he was due to pick up.

"I don't have it yet Georgie," she explained, "but as

PART ONE: TOIL

soon as I get it this afternoon, I will give you a ring"
"Okay," replied Georgie, "I'll be in the other office"
By 'the other office' he meant their local pub and Jackie had rung it so many times (because they didn't have a mobile phone between them) that the landlady wouldn't even bother telling Georgie she was on the other end of the line and would write down the serial number herself, which she then gave to either Bobbie or Georgie. When Jackie would ring the pub, she always put the phone on loud speaker so we could all hear what was going on in the background and it wasn't unusual to hear 'Knees Up Mother Brown' or some Max Bygraves classic being played on the piano as the customers sang along, all out of tune.

I would always have two phones on me plus this little plastic clip-on box thing that vibrated because at that time, we didn't have built-in vibrating phones. One of them was a standard mobile while the other was for internal use only and was connected to the offices above, which meant I could be contacted at any point throughout the day, even if I was sat on the bleedin' lavvy! John and Jackie and this young bloke called Tony who also worked upstairs in the main office, had by now discovered that I was well into my films and just say they were having a conversation on the phone to someone in Scotland and that conversation then diverted to a film question, they would always ring me down on the shop floor for the answer. I could be driving one of the forklifts at full speed one handed, to try and get a lorry loaded as quickly as possible and with the other hand, I'd be holding the phone and telling

BIPOLAR.....MAYBE?
(Volume Two)

them the answer to a question they had asked me. It got to such a stage that if people were having an argument about a film anywhere in the country, they would ring up and ask to be put through directly to me and therefore cut out the middle man or in Jackie's case, woman.

I have got a pretty deep voice (I don't mean my voice is pretty as in good looking... how could you have a good-looking voice? But rather, quite a deep voice) that is a bit gravelly sounding too, but I never used to be like that. Of course it wasn't deep when I was a kid but even when my voice broke, it still wasn't what you'd describe as very deep and I can actually remember the very day it changed for good. I was living in Chingford in London with Debbie and our two boys (Nin wasn't born yet) and my mum and dad came round to visit. They said that Patsy (my dad's brother) had rung them and asked if they wanted to go for a drink in Theydon Bois, where we used to live years ago. My mum and dad asked if me and Debbie wanted to go too but because we couldn't get a baby sitter, Debbie had to stay behind while I went with them to meet Patsy and my aunt Rosie. I had given up smoking for three years and a few months before that evening with my mum and dad and Patsy and Rosie, I had stupidly started up again. I was keen not to go back on the Benson and Hedges again as they were quite high in tar and so I switched to Silk Cut which only contained 5mg. After smoking them for a few weeks I changed to Silk Cut Low that contained 3mg of tar and a short while later, to Silk Cut Ultra that only contained 0.1mg. So low

where they in tar, the cigarette kept going out and I had to keep lighting it up again. Whereas Silk Cut were known as the main brand when it came to lower tar cigarettes, it has completely changed now with all the other brands getting in on the act and I couldn't tell you which was which because I switched to roll ups about four years ago. Anyway, it was while I was smoking Silk Cut Ultra when we went to the pub to see Patsy and Rosie and just before we left our house, my voice dropped considerably and has been that way ever since.
"What's happened to your voice?" Debbie asked.
"I dunno… I haven't even got a cold or anything"
All I can put it down to is I dragged so hard on those fucking cigarettes in order to try and get something out of them, they altered my voice and that was nearly twenty years ago.
I invited my friend Richard, who I'd known since I was four and still lived in Theydon, to come along and when we got to the pub, my uncle and aunt were already there and it was the first time that any of us had noticed Patsy was showing the early signs of Alzheimer's. Richard asked me what was wrong with my voice and I replied, "I think it's these fucking cigarettes"
He picked up the packet and after reading the information on the side he said, "0.1mg of tar! What is the fucking point? You might as well not smoke anything at all!"
"I know, I know but I'm finding it so hard to give up this time. I must admit that they are shit though and am gonna start smoking something a bit stronger"
Patsy then stood up and went off to the toilet as we were talking and he was gone for ages.

BIPOLAR…..MAYBE?
(Volume Two)

"Where's Patsy?" asked my mum and I told her I would go and look for him.

As I walked into the toilets, I saw him just standing there in the middle of the room.

"Are you alright Patsy?" I asked.

"Er… yeh, yeh… alright John," he replied and I could tell he couldn't find the exit.

"Come on mate," I said without making a big thing of it, "It's this way," and opened the door for him to walk back into the bar.

He immediately turned left but our table was to the right, so I gently held his arm and guided him to where we were all sitting. Rosie didn't say anything and just looked down at her glass but we all knew what was wrong. The worrying thing was, he drove to the pub and was going to drive home again but for the rest of the evening, he started to improve slightly. When it was time to go, we all got in our own cars (apart from Richard who walked home) and I could see the concern on my mum and dad's faces as Patsy drove away. I didn't see him again for another two years and when I did, the transformation was truly shocking.

Anyway, back to the deep voice.

B&Q's logistic department (or distribution centre) was where we would arrange for their transport to collect an order of pasting tables, which would fill a forty-foot or forty-five-foot trailer. Their forty five foot trailers were becoming increasingly common because they could obviously hold more products, which meant less lorries having to drive to their suppliers, which in turn meant a saving on fuel. That was fine by us because we were selling more pasting tables (an extra hundred on each

PART ONE: TOIL

load) and I would regularly ring logistics to arrange a pick-up time for a particular order. A girl called Suzie usually answered the phone and after a short while, we built up a good rapport between us and we'd always have a bit of a laugh or joke. On one occasion, she was being all flirty and said, "I've always liked your voice John… it's so sexy!"

I could see her imagining some six-foot-five, dark haired stud on the other end of the line and I answered, "Yeh… it's all the cigarettes and booze I get through each day"

The other end of the line went all quiet and I could tell her illusion had just been shattered. In an instant, I went from being a deep voiced Adonis to some old git who coughed his lungs up each morning, with a roll up hanging out the side of his mouth.

"So that's tomorrow at 14:30 hours," she finally said in an abrupt and authoritative tone before hanging up on me.

"Er… yeh," I said to no one… "Cheers," and then went into the tea room for a good old smoke.

Most of the hand-held tools on the factory floor were run by compressed air that ran down plastic tubing spiralled up to metal pipes, which in turn ran along the roof space to the main compressor near the far end of the building. If anyone was caught using these tools in an inappropriate manner (basically, firing them at each other) then it was an instant dismissal. There was one kid assembling wooden legs that had a strip of hardboard connecting each of them and they were joined together by four staples on either side of the hardboard. Earlier in the day I had to tell him to get on with his work because he wouldn't stop talking to this other kid standing close by to him and as I walked away I heard him say, "I fucking hate that cunt!"

Now I shouldn't have taken that personally even though it was directed at me, but I just couldn't help it. I was often more than fair with the workforce and was always willing to give someone a second chance but had to admit, what he said really got to me. Anyway, I did walk away and he got on with his work while I went over to where the heavy-duty tables were constructed, to see if an order I was waiting for was ready yet. While I was talking to the guy in charge of that department, I heard someone laughing out loud over by the main production line and looking over in that direction, I saw the kid who'd been making the legs, firing his staple gun at someone on the nailing machine. He then started to fan the gun with his left hand to emulate somebody out of a western and that's when I heard him cry out in pain. Rushing back over there, I saw this kid looking as white as a sheet with his hands held tightly together.

"What's the matter?" I asked him as he walked slowly towards me while staring down at his hands.

"A staple has gone into my thumb and I think I've hit a vein," he replied while looking paler and paler by the second.

"Let me have a look," I said as he slowly removed his right hand from his left.

The staple had gone as far as it could with the two end prongs protruding half an inch out of the front of the thumb, just below the nail with a small amount of blood around each prong. The joined end of the staple appeared to be imbedded into the back of his thumb and if the compressed air had been turned up any higher, I'm sure the entire staple would have gone right the way through and out of the other side.

"I don't think you've gone through a vein," I explained, "because you'd know about it if you had. The blood would be pumping out of the two holes"

"What…like this?" he said and squeezed the end of his thumb.

Two thin jets of blood shot ten feet into the air then stopped immediately when he let go, before he squeezed it again with the same outcome.

"Er yeh….pretty much like that," I replied, "You'd better come upstairs to get it looked at"

This kid was usually really cocky with plenty to say for himself but as we walked into the main office, he looked over to Fred who was sat behind the dispatch desk and said, "Fred… I've had an accident," in a meek and mild voice.

We took him into the tea room and after seeing the thumb, Fred went and fetched a pair of thin pliers. I held his hand facing palm upwards while Fred pushed the ends of the pliers deep against the back of the thumb.

"Aaaarrrggghhh! What are you doing?" cried the poor little lamb and then in an instant, Fred pulled the whole staple out in one go as I applied some cotton wool and a bandage.

As far as Fred knew, it had been an accident and he told the kid to go back downstairs and get on with his work because only one hand was needed to operate the staple gun. I then walked down the stairs with him and asked, "How are you feeling?"

BIPOLAR…..MAYBE?
(Volume Two)

"Not too bad, thank you John," he replied softly.

"Ah… that's good. Oh… and guess what"

"What's that John?" he asked as we reached the bottom of the stairs close to the main front door.

"You're sacked!"

"What? Why? Who… me?"

"Yep… you," I replied as I opened the exit door and led him outside.

"Why am I sacked?"

"For thinking you were Billy the Kid. Goodbye," and with that I shut the door, leaving him stood outside.

Now I'll be honest, I may have given him one more chance depending how he'd behaved in the past, but the main reason I sacked him wasn't for firing the stable gun all over the place, but for calling me a cunt. I know that's not professional and I should have been thicker skinned but hey ho…. that's that.

PART ONE: TOIL

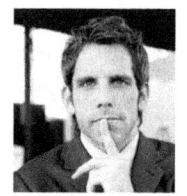

CHAPTER 5

On Tony's desk up in the main office, sat the absentee book which had to be filled in every time one of the work-force rang up with their excuse (I mean reason) for not coming in. Nine times out of ten you would have to ring them because they would hardly ever bother to call or leave a message and by far the main group of workers to have the most time off, were the school leavers. We'd be expected to write down in the book what they said their reasons for not coming in were, and me, John, Jackie and Tony would write down exactly, word for word, what they told us because some of the things they said were so funny.

I knew Simon thought we weren't taking things seriously but anyway, here are just a few examples of their explanations:

'I was riding into work on my bike, when both the wheels fell off and I broke my arms and legs. Should be back tomorrow'

'I lost my glasses and couldn't find my way into work. Still searching for them'

BIPOLAR…..MAYBE?
(Volume Two)

'I was staring at the ground and trying not to tread on the cracks in the pavement when I walked into a tree. Knocked myself out!'

Father talking about his son: 'His pet budgie George was taken seriously ill in the middle of the night and Gary had to rush him to the vet. He's still there now, waiting for George to come out of the operating theatre'

'My stars said to beware of Wednesday, so I thought it best if I stayed at home in bed where nothing can happen to me'

'I was running along because I was so keen to get to work and tripped over my laces. Went to hospital and they told me not to come in because I've broken two of my ribs'

'I was gonna come in with my mate but I fell down the stairs and squashed the cat'

'I've got the shits, stuck on bog!'

'My brother was bringing me in to work and drove over an old lady. At police station sorting it all out'

PART ONE: TOIL

'I forgot to wake up'

'Thought someone was following me so I hid behind a brick wall for two hours. Not worth coming in now'

'Had to bury my friend's squashed cat and I'm too upset to come into work today. Should be feeling much better by tomorrow'

'I swallowed a wasp and it's stinging the inside of my belly. My mum says I have to stay at home and drink lots of water so it will drown it'

'Hit my head and lost my memory. Who are you?'

'Watched a horror film last night and I'm too scared to come in to work. I will watch a funny film tonight and will feel much better in the morning'

'Can't come in today because my mum says I have to tidy my bedroom'

'Fell down a manhole. Too upset to come in'

BIPOLAR…..MAYBE?
(Volume Two)

'A firework came in through my window and set my bed on fire. Got to go shopping for a new bed'

'Caught the flu off my mum. She's better now but I'm in a right old state. Won't be in for ages'

'I got mugged by the pizza delivery man. Got no money for a pizza or the bus into work'

'Had a nose bleed for six hours, scared I'm gonna run out of blood so best to stay at home with cotton wool up my nostrils'

They were all clearly taking the piss but nevertheless, I had to admire their imagination and I really wish I'd photocopied them all because there were some absolute classics, but unfortunately, I didn't and can only remember those few examples.

A middle aged guy called Peter started working for us and at first I thought he'd be quite capable because he was well spoken and seemed to pay full attention as I explained how to operate one of the staple guns. Like the kid who shot his thumb, Peter was working on the paste table legs and after seeing that he could do it properly and watching him for several minutes, I got called away to another part of the factory. About ten minutes later, I walked back to the production line and

could see Fred having a go at Peter.
"Not like that!" yelled Fred, "Hold the gun like this"
He'd been doing it absolutely fine when I was with him and I can only assume he had changed the way I'd told him to hold the gun when I walked away.
"You don't have to shout at me," he said to Fred.
"I wouldn't have to if you fucking did it right!" and with that, Peter started walking to the exit while calling out, "I've never been spoken to like that before… you haven't heard the last of this!"
Three days later, I was outside closing the two big wooden gates in the loading area after a B&Q lorry had just pulled away, and I saw Peter walking along on the pavement. As he came past the gates I called out, "Hiya Pete, how are you doing?"
Not looking at me, he continued to march along and without stopping or turning around he called out, "You'll be hearing from my barrister in due course!"
Fucking nutcase!

At the end of each month, a magazine devoted to all thing's woodwork (how exciting!) came in the post and for me, the most interesting part (but also the most gruesome) was on the very last page where it featured terrible injuries caused by some pretty lethal machinery to the person operating them. It should have been titled 'Injury of the Month' and there was one in particular that still makes me shudder when I think about it. This guy was cutting sheets of chipboard on a band saw and the hand pushing them was positioned just like Mr. Spock's four fingered Vulcan salute, with the thumb outstretched and the middle and ring finger parted so the hand formed a V shape. Something must have distracted him because instead of moving his hand to the side of the chipboard so it was out of the way of the rotating band saw, he kept it in the same position and carried on pushing. The razor sharp teeth of the saw began to tear their way into the fleshy part of skin in between the parted four fingers, as easily as a hot knife through butter. Such was the force that he'd been pushing the chipboard, the band saw continued cutting into the hand itself and by the time a work colleague had rushed over and switched the machine off, the saw had cut all the way down to his wrist… nasty!

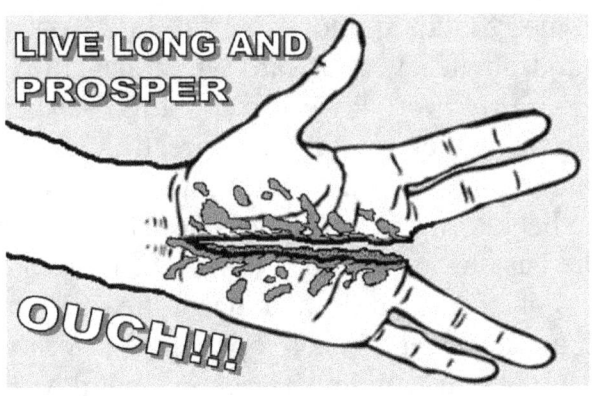

One of our electric forklifts was playing up one time and so we called a service engineer who came in to take a look at it. I drove the forklift outside when he arrived and made him a cup of tea and after he'd sorted the problem out, he started telling me about some of the accidents people had suffered while driving them. The masts on modern forklifts are designed in such a way that the driver is able to see through them, with the hydraulic powered cylinder lifting up out of the way

PART ONE: TOIL

with the forks. Directly under the cylinder is a thick metal bar keeping it in place and joins both sides of the mast pillars for added strength. This metal bar rises up and down with the hydraulic cylinder and forks and lowers down to just a few inches off the ground. A second set of mast pillars sit inside the outer pair and run along on wheels set inside a greased track on each outer pillar. It's on this second set that the hydraulic cylinder and forks are attached and the service guy told me about this bloke who noticed some cardboard stuck inside one of the greased tracks while the forks were up in the air. He leant forward so his head and arm were sticking through the outer mast in order to try and remove the cardboard and as he did, his chest pushed the up and down lever forward which began to lower the forks. However, lowering the forks also meant lowering the thick metal bar directly beneath the hydraulic cylinder and as a result, it came into contact with the back of his head. He was now trapped and the more the bar pushed his head down, the more pressure it put on his chest, which also meant the forks and bar carried on lowering. When operating a forklift, no matter how hard you push the up and down lever forward, the forks will only go down at a certain speed, which isn't that fast, so this poor bloke must have been fully aware what was about to happen to him. The thick metal bar slowly pushed his head further down until his face came into contact with a second bar that is in a fixed position just below the dashboard of the forklift. There was absolutely nothing this guy could do and as the two bars got closer and closer together, they acted like some sort of blunt guillotine but instead of the blades decapitating him in the blink of an eye, the blunt lumps of metal slowly began to crush his skull until they finally ripped the top of his head off. It must have been an awful sight with brains, blood and bone all over the place and the forks would have carried on lowering until they couldn't go any further… gruesome!

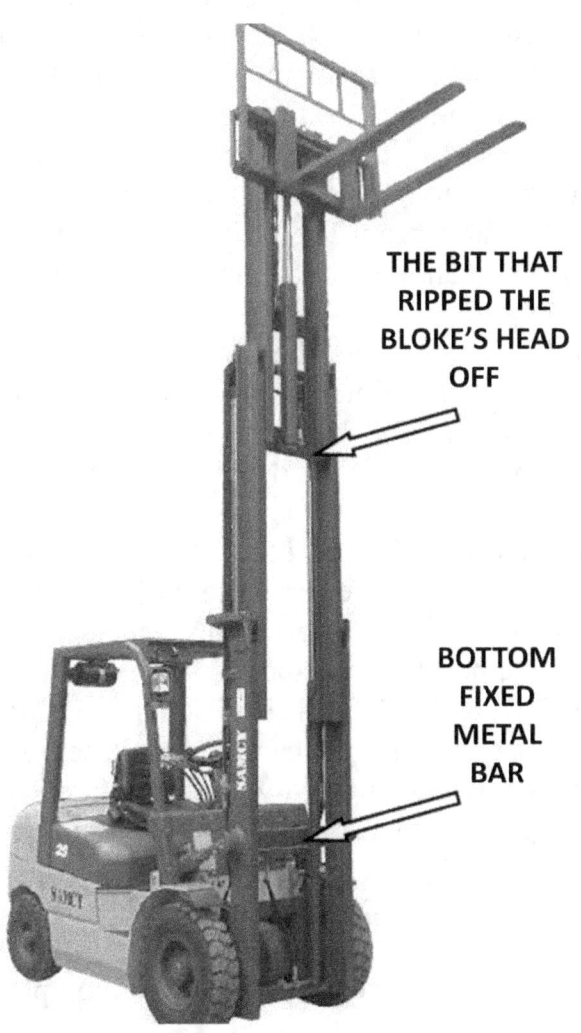

PART ONE: TOIL

All this talk of hideous accidents puts me in mind of my friend Ed's dad Ray who was backing a lorry into their waste paper yard. He made sure he was stood at such an angle so the driver could see him in his wing mirror and kept on motioning him to reverse with his left arm while slowly walking backwards at the same time. For some reason, he wanted the lorry undercover inside the building itself and as it backed towards the rear wall, Ray held his hand out with the palm facing the lorry to indicate for it to come to stop. What he failed to notice however was that the lorry had reversed closer to himself, which now meant the driver could no longer see him in his mirror. The back of the lorry touched Ed's dad's hand and continued to slowly roll backwards.

"Whoa!" yelled Ray but the driver couldn't hear him owing to the noise of machinery operating nearby.

"Whoa!" repeated Ray but again the lorry continued to reverse while pushing Ed's dad's arm back at the same time.

It was then that Ray could feel his elbow touch something and when he turned to see what it was, he could see his arm was pinned against a metal post which helped to support the roof above.

"WHOA! WHOA! STOP THE FUCKING LORRY!"

It was no use, the driver clearly couldn't hear him and now Ray's arm was trapped with the palm of his hand pushed against the back of the lorry and his elbow up against the metal post. The driver was only doing 1mph which made what was about to happen, all the more eye watering. Millimetre by millimetre, the lorry ever so slowly rolled backwards, with the driver completely

BIPOLAR…..MAYBE?
(Volume Two)

oblivious and millimetre by millimetre, Ray's arm began to crush between the two solid objects. The lorry continued to reverse for six inches, causing Ray's forearm to crush six inches shorter in length and he must have been totally aware of his radius and ulna bones snapping like twigs, with the disconnected ends pushing against the skin and deforming the arm. The driver only stopped when he could feel some resistance and must have figured that the back of the lorry was touching the wall.

When I was a kid, I always noticed that Ray's arm was deformed and when I asked Ed why, he relayed the horrific story I've just shared with you. I never had the guts to ask his dad myself because he seemed to be such a surly person and definitely had a temper on him, but that doesn't lessen the impact of that terrible tale. Man, that must have been painful!

PART ONE: TOIL

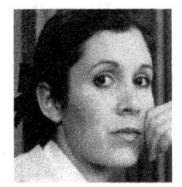

CHAPTER 6

Wednesday, 13th February 2002
We had a new kid start called Stephen, who was about eighteen and had down syndrome. I wasn't particularly happy about this because the forklifts were constantly rushing about, in and out of the building and I felt that kind of environment would be very dangerous for him. Stephen was on some kind of work experience program however which meant he was free labour and so any concerns I might have had, went right out the window and I spent most of the day checking he was okay. Just after lunchtime on that day, I couldn't find anything for him to do that I'd considered to be safe and so I gave him a dustbin and a broom and asked him to sweep up, outside in the yard. We were trying to get an order of heavy-duty tables finished by three o'clock because a lorry was due to come and collect them, and so I forgot all about Stephen until after I'd loaded up the truck with the forklift. Once the driver had gone and I'd shut the main gates, I went back into the factory and lifted a pack of fifteen foot timber with the side loader, onto a scissor lift which fed the planer. When that was done, I climbed down off the side loader and saw Stephen

standing close by, with the handle of the broom held firmly in each hand but no sign of the dustbin.

"Alright Stephen," I said after walking up to him, "Where's your bin?"

He thought for a moment before replying, "I've been here," and with that I burst out laughing.

I'm sure he didn't mean it to sound like a joke but the timing was absolutely perfect and I could see the look of confusion on his face as if to say, "What's so funny?"

He stood there for a while saying nothing before eventually coming out with, "John?"

I could tell he wanted something and replied, "Yeeeeh?"

"Would I be able to take some wood home tonight, I want to make a model aeroplane"

"Oh is that all," I said, "Yes of course… I'll sort you something out when it's time to go home," and with that, a big smile came over his face and he went off in search of the dustbin.

I was on the forklift shortly afterwards, loading another lorry when my internal phone rang.

"Hello?" I said.

"Hi John… its Jackie," came the reply, "Your mum is on the phone"

"Oh right…. cheers Jackie," I answered and wondered what my mum wanted because she never rang me when I was at work.

"Hi John," came the voice on the other end of the line.

"Hi mum… is everything okay?"

"Patsy died a short while ago"

Although I knew he was very ill and it was just a matter of time, it still came as a shock.

PART ONE: TOIL

"John...are you there?"
"Er... yeh mum, thanks for letting me know"
Along with Michael's dad Ernie, Patsy was definitely one of my favourite uncles on my dad's side of the family and after hanging up, I still continued to load the lorry but couldn't stop thinking about him for the rest of the day. A couple of months earlier, I had been driving on the M25 and was just about to get off at the Waltham Abbey junction to make my way home on the Epping New Road. Patsy and Rosie lived in Waltham Abbey and just as I reached the roundabout at the bottom of the junction, instead of taking the third exit which would have taken me home, I turned left and decided to pay them both a visit. Rosie opened the door and seemed surprised to see me and after inviting me in, she took me to the living room where Patsy was sitting in a chair watching the television. Actually, to say he was watching the T.V isn't the right description because he was just staring at it and didn't seem to comprehend what was on the screen, which for some reason, I'll always remember was Thunderbirds. Rosie went into the kitchen to make me a cup of tea and while she was out of the room, I walked over to Patsy and placed my hand on top of his. There was absolutely no sign he even knew I was there and he continued to stare straight ahead. One of his favourite films was 'The Outlaw Josey Wales' and he always used to say, "I generally watch that a couple of times a week"

"Have you watched it recently?" I asked, knowing full well he wouldn't answer me, but I was trying to get him to remember something... anything.

Nothing...no response whatsoever and after repeating

BIPOLAR.....MAYBE?
(Volume Two)

the question several times and describing some of the bits in the film, I gave up and sat back down on the sofa. Rosie came in with the tea and some biscuits and after placing the tray on the coffee table, she took Patsy's cup and placed it on the armrest of his chair before positioning his fingers through the handle so he was holding it. There was no way he was going to lift it to his mouth and as Rosie sat down next to me she said, "I always do that but he never drinks it… you never know though, he might do one day"

The last time I had seen Patsy and Rosie was a couple of years earlier when me, my mum and dad and my mate Richard went to the pub in Theydon Bois (I mentioned it earlier) That was the time when we all noticed the early signs of his dementia and it was such a shock to see him now, sitting in his armchair, totally oblivious to his surroundings. Me and Rosie were quietly talking about that time when all of a sudden Patsy yelled out, "You fucking cunt!" before falling silent again. We both burst out laughing because it came from nowhere but at the same time, it was so sad to see him like that.

So there I was on the forklift, loading up the lorry with the news of his death constantly on my mind. I started to think back to the time before he was ill and when I'd finally finished loading the lorry, I couldn't stop laughing to myself.

"What's so funny?" asked the driver.

"Oh it's nothing, I'm just thinking about something," I replied.

Patsy always dressed smartly for work, with a shirt and tie and would constantly polish his shoes by rubbing

PART ONE: TOIL

them on the back of his trouser legs. Maybe that was the early signs of his Alzheimer's, who knows but as the years went by, he started to do it more often and would also talk increasingly quicker, like he was nervous or something. We would get our lunches from the bakers up the road and on one occasion, Patsy asked for a steak and kidney pie. While the rest of us started tucking into our grub with unwashed hands, Patsy got a tea chest and turned it upside down before placing a tea towel over it like a table cloth. He then got a chair and sat down by the tea chest with his own personal knife and fork in hand and a paper napkin tucked into the collar of his shirt. The pie was baking hot so he cut it in half in order for it to cool down slightly and then took a big mouthful. As he sat there chewing contently on the pie, he gazed down at the rest of it sitting on the tea chest and then a concerned expression appeared on his face. He moved his head closer to the meat pie and although none of us knew what was the matter with him, we were all laughing at the way he'd set up his 'dining table' and the paper napkin etc. He stared closer still at the pie before a look of horror came over his face and all of a sudden he yelled out, "Whaaaaaarrrrgghh!" with bits of chewed steak and kidney pie being spat out of his mouth in all directions. He then pulled the paper napkin out of his collar and spat the rest of the pie he'd been eating into it before standing up and rushing into the toilets. We could all hear noises like he was being sick and Michael stood up and walked over to the rest of the uneaten pie. Upon closer inspection, he burst out laughing and so we all went to have a look too. There was a huge bluebottle fly amongst the meat but what

BIPOLAR…..MAYBE?
(Volume Two)

made it funnier was that only half was left, which meant Patsy had eaten the other half. My nephew Lee's mate called Simon Osbourne (or Oz as everybody called him) had just started working for us at this point and we gave him the list of lunches required each day and asked him to go and get them for us.

"Aren't you going to give me any money?" he asked Michael.

"No… that's alright," replied Mick, "Just tell them to put it on our account"

"Oh, okay then," said Oz and went off on his merry way.

So, when he was given all the lunches, the lady said, "That will be twelve pounds please," and Oz smiled back at her and replied, "Can you put it on our account?"

The lady's happy mood changed to anger in a split second and she said, "What bleedin' account? You haven't got an account!" and with that, Oz had to make his way back to the factory to get the money we should have given him in the first place.

"I felt like a right fucking idiot," he said as we all burst out laughing.

Roy was the person who usually operated the gluing machine, where cartons were fed into it and the rollers slowly moved the carton through the machine, applying a thin line of glue onto the end flap. He couldn't have been in on this particular day and so Patsy fed each carton into the machine. As per usual, he was wearing the obligatory shirt and tie and he must have leant too far forward because his tie got caught in the rollers and slowly started to drag his head closer and closer to the revolving wheels (of death!)

"Help me!" he screamed out, "I'm being strangled alive!"

By trying to keep his head away from the machine, his tie was tightening around his neck and it was choking him, resulting in his face turning bright red with a hint of purple.

"Help me somebody!" he pleaded and trying not to laugh, I went over and pressed the emergency stop button, with his face only two inches away from the rollers.

It was like something out of a Batman episode where Robin was being dragged into a machine and Batman had to save him, but you had to wait until the next week to find out what happened. I had to get a pair of scissors and cut his beloved tie to set him free and then lifted his collar so I could just about get one of the scissor blades between what was left of the tie and the collar, before cutting that away too.

The office at A. Barrett & Sons had cartons stacked on top of it and on another occasion, Patsy leant a metal ladder against it and started climbing up so he could get to some of the boxes. He got to the top of the ladder and was holding onto the highest rung with both his hands while his feet were stood on the forth rung down. Just as he was about to climb onto the roof, the bottom of the ladder slipped outwards on the smooth floor whilst the top of it slid down the side of the office wall. This happened during tea break, so we were all sat there watching the whole thing, which happened in an instant and what made it look so funny was that both his hands were still held on tight to the top rung. The ladder slid all the way down the wall and ended up flat on the floor, trapping Patsy's hands underneath so he couldn't move. Mick had to go and lift the end of the ladder slightly so Patsy could get his hands out and after getting up on his feet, he ran round in circles, holding both hands under his armpits while biting the collar of his shirt, which was a thing he always did if he was upset about something. I noticed as the years passed by, Patsy doing that more and more often and just by being the person he was, I reckon that had a lot to do with his later dementia. Him and Rosie lived about three miles away from my mum and dad at the time and they were just about to go out to the shops one Saturday afternoon, when Patsy noticed the top step on their staircase had a squeak when stood upon.

"I'm just gonna take a quick look at this Rose," he told my aunt.

"Come on Palla (his nickname) we won't get to the shops at this rate," she replied.

"It won't take a minute," he said while ripping the carpet off the step.

"Oh fucking hell," he mumbled under his breath.

"What's wrong?" asked Rosie.

"It's chipboard and the nails are right the way in"

"Just leave it for now and look at it when we get back"

"No, it's alright… I'll just go and get a screwdriver and a hammer from the garage and try and dig the end of the nails out"

"Don't you go ruining our staircase," she said as he walked past her and made his way to the garage.

At that point, the phone rang and it was their youngest daughter, Eileen.

"I wasn't sure if you said you were going shopping," she said to her mum.
"We're supposed to be but he's got the carpet up and messing around with the staircase"
"What's the matter?"
"With what… the staircase or him?"
"The staircase"
"Oh, I don't know, he reckons there's a squeak but I've never noticed it"
BANG! BANG! BANG! BANG!
"What's that noise?" asked Eileen.
"That's him sodding around with a bleedin' hammer"
BANG! BANG! BANG! BANG!
"What did you say?"
BANG! BANG! BANG! BANG!
"It's him and a hammer"
BANG! BANG! BANG! BANG! "Oh fucking hell!"
"What's going on up there?" yelled Rosie.
"I've just whacked my fingers with the hammer"
"What did he just say?" asked Eileen.
"He's just whacked his fingers with the hammer"
"You'll never get to the shops at this rate"
"Don't I know it. Palla…. Eileen says we'll never get to the shops at this rate!"
"Tell her to mind her own business!"
"What did he just say mum?"
"He said he won't be too long"
"Why is he trying to get the step up? Surely if it's squeaking he needs to screw it down tighter"
"Hold on, I'll ask him. Eileen says, why are you trying to get the step up instead of screwing it down?"
"I've nearly got all the nails out now!"

BIPOLAR…..MAYBE?
(Volume Two)

"Hurry up!"
"Shut your face!" There you are, I've done it!"
"Well?"
"There's nothing under here that would make it squeak… only a water pipe but that's not touching the step"
"Well put it all back again and do what Eileen said, by screwing it down"
So, Patsy went back to the garage and got a load of screws and a screw gun before returning to the top step.
"It's gone quiet," said Eileen, "What's he up to?"
WHIIIIIRRRR, WHIIIIIRRRR, WHIIIIIRRRR!
"He's screwing it down like you said"
"There you are, all done!" said Patsy with a smile on his face as he walked down the stairs into the living room where Rosie was on the phone.
"Does that mean we can go to the shops now?" she asked.
"We can do if you get off the bleedin' phone! I'm just gonna put this stuff back in the garage"
"Okay… I'll get our coats out from under the stairs.
"Alright then mum," said Eileen, "I'll let you go. Pop in on your way back," and with that she hung up.
Rosie made her way to the cupboard under the stairs to get their coats as Patsy was pulling down the garage door.
"AAAAARRRGGGHH!" she screamed.
"What's happened?" yelled Patsy as he came running back into the house.
"Look at my hair," she sobbed, "its ringing wet!"
"How did that happen?"
"There's water pouring through the ceiling in the

cupboard under the stairs!"
Patsy was quiet for a moment as he was trying to figure out what had happened before finally replying, "I must have screwed through the water pipe. It's all that Eileen's fault, I'll bloody kill her!"

A load of us went to the villa in Portugal one time and Patsy, Rosie, their eldest daughter Suzie and her husband Eddie came out after we'd been there for a week. We had such a great time because there were loads of us, including my mate Richard and my sister Jane's friend Denise too. It was August and the heat was almost unbearable but Patsy being Patsy, he wore a suit with a shirt and tie done up to the neck when we went out for meals in the evening, even though the temperature had only dropped slightly. Eddie was into all that keep fit malarkey at the time and would run along the dirt track that surrounded the villas during the daytime. It must have been about a mile long and Patsy thought, "I'm having some of that," so decided to do the run for himself.

The sun was at its strongest and beat down on him as he struggled along the track and about half way round, he collapsed in a heap on the ground. Luckily, Eddie had been running at the same time and must have looked behind him when he couldn't hear Patsy running any more. He had to virtually carry him back to the villa and the only sympathy he got from the rest of us was the sound of hysterical laughter as he lay out flat on the marble floor, next to the swimming pool.

Before Lee started to work for us, both Patsy and my dad were the lorry drivers at Barrett's and even at a

BIPOLAR.....MAYBE?
(Volume Two)

young age during my school holidays when I went into work, I could see just how good they were. I used to love going out with Patsy because he was always happy and would whistle away to himself as he held the steering wheel all dainty, much like Oliver Hardy. He was one of those blokes who everyone knew and liked and I was definitely part of that category.

I remember going into work with my dad on one occasion and we were stuck in traffic in Forest Road which led into Walthamstow from the Waterworks roundabout. The particular part of Forest Road we were stuck in had two lanes on either side and my dad's lorry was on the inside lane because we wanted to go straight ahead at the traffic lights and the outer lane was designated for turning right only. Our lane was hardly moving whereas the outer one was moving pretty steadily and as we were stuck there, a motorbike was trying to get out of a small turning on our left. He wanted to cross both our lanes and turn right so he'd be heading in the other direction and even though my dad had about four car lengths of space in front of him, he waited so the motorbike could get out. This is how clever my dad was: He could tell the bike rider couldn't see what was coming in the outer lane to our right and because traffic was moving in that particular lane, my dad put his right indicator on.

"How comes you want to get in that lane?" I asked.

"I don't," replied my dad, "but by putting my indicator on, it will stop the traffic coming past us and they will hopefully let me in"

"But you said you didn't want to go in that lane"

"I don't but when someone stops, I'll let the bloke on

PART ONE: TOIL

the motorbike know that it's safe to pull out"
I remember thinking, "Wow… I would never have thought of that (although now I'd class myself in pretty much the same league as my dad and Patsy) and that's something they don't teach you when you're learning"
My dad could hardly read or write but would constantly surprise me just how smart he was.

So back to Simon's place and I'd just finished loading the lorry with the forklift whilst reminiscing about Patsy, and right at that point, the five o'clock bell went and all the workforce started to clock out. As I was about to go upstairs and get the paperwork for the driver to sign, I saw Stephen (the guy with Down syndrome) carrying one of the fifteen-foot-long pieces of timber I'd put onto the scissor lift a couple of hours earlier.
"Hold on," I called out, "Where are you going with that?"
"You said I could take a piece of wood home to make a model aeroplane"
"Yeh… a piece of wood, not a whole fucking length of it! Anyway, how did you intend to get that home?"
"My dad has come to get me in his car"
"He only drives a mini and you'd need a bloody lorry to get that home! Put it back and I'll sort you out a few off cuts"
"Okay then!" he replied and took the wood back from where he'd got it.

Patsy's funeral was on the 22nd of February 2002 and during the service, I started to cry because I loved that man and couldn't believe he was actually dead. When we all got back to Rosie's house, Suzie (their daughter) came up to me and said, "You're soft hearted ain't you John"

"Er yeh," I replied, "I never used to get upset like that but I've changed somehow"

"It doesn't matter," she said, "I think it's good to show your emotions"

"I've started to learn that now," I said, "and couldn't care less what other people think"

PART ONE: TOIL

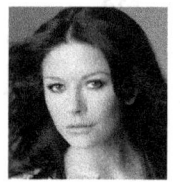

CHAPTER 7

I wrote in 'Volume One' about a guy called Beige who worked at Simon's place and was one of the Bethnal Green group that came in on the minibus. His main role was as foreman on the shop floor and he had such a quiet way about him which I really respected. Beige wasn't his real name (that was Anthony) and it only came about because he was from Barbados and thinking about it now, it sounds racist but it never seemed to bother him and I always felt it sounded pretty cool. I would talk to him a lot at lunchtimes, where he would eat in a small cabin constructed for him on the factory floor and he always told me when he retired, he wanted to move back to Barbados. Personally I thought he must be completely bonkers living in this country with our crappy weather but like he said, he was eighteen years old when he emigrated to England and at that time, there just wasn't that much work available in his home country. I really hoped he would one day manage to get back to Barbados and enjoy his retirement in the sun and he said that when he did eventually get back there, I could go and visit him. Me, Debbie and the boys went to Barbados in late December 2000 and I suppose strictly speaking, Nin went too even though she was still inside her mum's tummy. When I told Beige we were going, he told us to visit Bridgetown where he was born, which is also the capital city and I asked him which was the best rum to drink.

"John.... you must try Mount Gay Rum, she so smooth," he replied in his still distinctive accent.

"What I didn't tell him was that I planned to get him a bottle and when we got back and I gave it to him, he was genuinely grateful and delighted at the same time.

January 2004

It had been another freezing cold day at Simon's firm and that's the trouble when it comes to factories, no matter how much heating the building has installed, it just isn't enough to warm the place up. We had the same thing at Barrett's and it can literally feel like you're working in a freezer with the metal machinery as cold as ice on your hands. When I got home that night, I ran a hot bath and lay there for half an hour, letting the warmth of the water soak into my bones. Debbie came into the bathroom and sat down on the laundry box before asking, "Is everything okay?"

"Not really," I replied, "I've been working in factories for over twenty years now and just can't do it anymore"

"What do you mean?" she asked.

"It's about time I did something else"

"But what else could you do? You don't have any qualifications"

She would always say that to our boys when they moaned about school and stressed how important it was to take their exams and study as hard as possible. The thing with me though was I knew when I left school, I

PART ONE: TOIL

was going straight into the family business and felt like I didn't need to take any exams, but in hindsight I knew I should have.

"Didn't you say the other day that your dad was getting pissed off with the guy who does his decorating?" I said.

Debbie's dad was a property developer who bought houses in a state of disrepair before renovating them and putting them back on the market in the hope of getting a decent profit.

"Who do you mean.... Martin?" she asked.

"I think that's his name.... yeh"

"He's absolutely hopeless.... my dad says he hardly ever turns up and when he does, he's always late"

"That's right, I remember you telling me about him," I said.

"Are you thinking you could do the decorating instead?"

"Why not? I can't be any worse than him"

"But I told you the other week that my dad is starting to wind down and hopefully retire at the end of the year"

"Yeh I know but what if we go halves with him on the next couple of houses and when he does retire, we should hopefully have enough money to go it alone"

Debbie thought for a while before finally answering, "But dad said things are starting to get more and more difficult and the profit margins aren't what they used to be"

"Yeh but you could still have a word with him and see what he says"

"I'm seeing him tomorrow and I'll have a word, but I think I know what his answer will be"

BIPOLAR…..MAYBE?
(Volume Two)

"That's why I suggested I do the decorating and help out with anything else"

"But if he does say it's not a good idea, then you will only have enough work until the end of the year"

"I know it's a risk but I really can't stand doing factory work anymore"

"Okay… I'll speak to him tomorrow when he comes round"

I spent the whole of the next day at Simon's place, thinking about the conversation between Debbie and her dad and couldn't wait to get home to see how it had gone. Although the overriding decision to quit was due to the fact I couldn't stand working in a factory any longer, I was also aware that over the course of the last year, things were beginning to change. Me and Simon had gone on a business trip to Poland the previous year to have meetings with our paste table suppliers and we stayed in this beautiful five star hotel that directly overlooked Piłsudski Square, with the Tomb of the Unknown Soldier clearly visible from our room. The tomb is constantly lit by an eternal flame and guarded by two soldiers from the Representative Battalion of the Polish Army, with the changing of the guard taking place on the hour of every hour daily and this happens 365 days a year. The first thing I noticed when we entered the lobby of the hotel, were several women sitting by themselves and they constantly looked up when anyone walked in. It was clear to me they were high class hookers wearing what looked like very expensive fur coats and I was surprised the management of the hotel allowed them to be there but

PART ONE: TOIL

I'm guessing the Polish culture must be different from ours. We had a meeting scheduled for the following morning with two of our suppliers but nothing for the rest of our first day and so after wolfing down a delicious à la carte meal, we decided to have a look round the old town and went into a couple of bars to wet our whistles and I don't mean suits.
(When I say the old town, there wasn't hardly much of it left because nearly 90% had been destroyed by the Germans in the second world war)
Our agent, who was the go between with us and our suppliers, met us in the hotel lobby at nine o'clock the next morning and said that the boss of our biggest supplier would be picking us up in half an hour and driving us to their factory. So, thirty minutes later, this guy who must have been in his late fifties and looking like a gangster, walked into the lobby, flanked by this tall and stocky younger bloke and an attractive girl who was probably in her mid-twenties. Our agent introduced us all to each other and after shaking hands with everyone, he explained that the girl and younger guy were the older man's children who both worked for him. The girl was the only one who could speak English out of the trio and she asked us if we would follow them outside, so they could drive us to the factory. It must have snowed heavily during the night and the sun's rays shone brilliantly off the carpet of white which covered everything. Their car was directly outside the main entrance of the hotel and the younger guy opened one of the back doors of this brand new, metallic grey, seven series BMW to let us in. Even though it was a big car it was still a bit of a squeeze, with me, our agent, the

daughter and Simon sat in the back whilst the dad did the driving and his son sat in the front passenger seat.

"Thank fuck he's sat in the front," I told myself because he was a big bloke and it would have been even more of a squeeze if he'd been in the back with us.

Although the drive was a little over three hours, it seemed to take for ever and I remember being surprised at just how many cars and lorries had slid off the main roads due to the snow and ended up lying in a field, because I thought they would have been used to such weather. Fred, Simon and Matthew had been considering buying a factory for themselves in Poland because the cost of producing pasting tables out there would have been significantly lower than in the U.K and our agent was due to take us to a couple of empty buildings the next day. The car journey dragged on for an eternity and the further we drove, the deeper we travelled into wooded areas until we finally arrived at our destination, which was right in the middle of a forest. We were shown around the production area and it was strange seeing these guys making paste tables much the same as our own work force but in a slightly different order. Whereas we would buy much of our timber in already cut to the width and depth required, this company bought in whole tree trunks (or just cut them down themselves from the forest) and after sawing them to size, they'd put the lengths of timber into shipping containers that had been converted into giant kilns. The timbers would stay in there for up to a week until they were fully dried out and then the rest of the manufacturing process would take place. There was another son on the shop floor who I guessed was the production manager and he, his brother and sister along with their dad, took us to this other building where the offices were housed, and behind them was a small warehouse which they took us to. Inside was a red Lamborghini, a black two door BMW convertible and a top of the range Suzuki motorbike, along with what looked like, brand new gym equipment, which the first son obviously used because he was built like a brick shit house. You could bet your life their work force hadn't seen all this stuff because they were probably paid peanuts, so that was obviously something they didn't want them to know about. There was something about these people I just didn't trust and if I had been them, the last thing I would have done was to show us the spoils of their profits because it meant they must have been overcharging us. To me this showed they couldn't care less what we thought and part of me was thinking, "They're gonna end up cutting out the middle man (being us) and start selling directly to our main customers"

A short while later, they took us out to lunch in this tiny village in the middle of nowhere and suggested we try their local delicacy which was some kind of brown watery soup with a whole, hard-boiled egg floating in the middle of it, but much to my surprise, it was quite nice. With the daughter translating to her father and then back to us and with the input from our agent as well, we arranged the next three months of deliveries and also discussed about the possibility of them producing some of our heavy duty tables as well. Personally, I thought this was a big mistake because it meant they had even more control over us and it could give them greater a reason to do away with us all together. By saying 'do away' I don't mean kill us but just by the looks on their faces, I wouldn't have put it past them; I mean cutting us out of the equation in a business sense. By the time they had taken us back to the hotel, it was dark outside and after a quick shower and something to eat, we went out to a couple of bars for a much needed drink.

The next morning, our agent was in the lobby at 9am on the dot and after we'd ordered some coffee, he took us to a couple of empty factories he thought we might be interested in. We drove south close to Krakow with the Karpaty Mountains visible in the distance and the first building he showed us was actually a set of three separate buildings but they seemed far too small to be of any interest to us.

"Don't worry," he said, "I think the next factory will be much more suitable," and with that, we all got back in his car and began to drive further into dense forest.

It took roughly an hour to reach our next destination and after pulling into a dirt track off of a B road, we stopped by a ranch style gate that had a man with a rifle strapped over his shoulder, standing next to it.

"What's with the gun?" asked Simon.

"Oh, it's nothing to worry about," laughed our agent, "he probably uses it for hunting rabbits and such like"

I looked over to Simon and neither of us seemed that convinced and why was he guarding the gate? The guy with the rifle then slowly opened the gate and waved to our agent as we drove through, before closing it again behind us. We travelled about another five hundred yards and after taking a sharp turn left, came upon this

PART ONE: TOIL

large stone building in front of us. Once we had parked up by the main entrance to the building, the man with the rifle came walking up to us and shook our hands before gesturing for us to follow him inside. Just as I was about to go in, I looked over to my left and saw a train track that ended close to the rear of the building, which had weeds and long lengths of grass growing between the sleepers. We entered the building, which was completely empty and I was convinced it must have been a concentration camp during the Second World War. As I mentioned before, the building seemed to be constructed out of large slabs of stone and as we walked around, I had an image of prisoners crammed inside, like sardines in a tin. Our agent had been correct when he said this building was much more suitable for our purposes but the thought of having to work there gave me the creeps.

As we drove back to Warsaw, we took a detour and paid a visit to another of our suppliers, whose premises were also set within a forest. The setup was very similar to the other supplier and when it was time for all the work force to go home, the boss suggested we go back to his home for something to eat. His house was set within the grounds of the factory and I remember being surprised just how small it was when we were greeted inside by his wife, who was holding their one-year-old daughter. She made us some snacks to munch on and after we'd finished eating, the husband poured us some Polish vodka and then went over to a cupboard and got three guns out. The first was a Glock 35 semi-automatic pistol which he held out straight in both hands and with one eye shut, aimed it around the room with his baby

BIPOLAR…..MAYBE?
(Volume Two)

daughter crawling on the floor. Me and Simon looked at each other as if to say, "Shit! We're in the middle of nowhere with this lunatic pointing a gun at us and his daughter!"

We had no idea if the thing was loaded or not as we fidgeted in our seats and the next gun he showed us was a .357 Magnum which he also waved around the room. In a strong Polish accent he said, "And finally, I want to show you….."

"We had better get going now," interrupted Simon, "It's getting late and there's a long journey back"

"Oh… okay," said the husband with a look of disappointment on his face and with that, we all stood up and made our way to the door.

The drive back seemed to take ages and because Simon couldn't be bothered to talk to the agent anymore for the rest of the evening, he pretended to be asleep in the back and left it all to me (the dirty rat!)

So going back to when I was lying in the bath talking to Debbie and how I could tell things weren't the same anymore at Simon's firm. B&Q was by far our biggest customer and they were putting more and more pressure on us to reduce the cost of out pasting tables. Combine that with our Polish suppliers who were sure to go straight to our customers directly and cut us out completely, I knew it was just a matter of time before the business would collapse.

"Did you speak to your dad?" I asked Debbie when I got home from work the following day.

"I did and he agreed it would be a good idea for you to do the decorating but said things were getting more and more difficult when it comes to finding houses to work on"

"Does that mean he doesn't think we should do it?"

"No.... he's just warning us that it's not so easy to find a suitable property because so many people are turning their hands to it and as a result, the profit margins aren't as great as they used to be"

"What do you think I should do?" I asked Debbie.

"It's your decision," she replied, "but if you think Simon's place is declining... then why not, you've got nothing to lose"

I spoke to Debbie's dad myself the following weekend and he reiterated what he'd told her and didn't rule the idea out, but was rather just warning me that the property developing side of things was becoming increasingly difficult.

"I think the main reason is all of these property development programmes popping up on the television," he explained, "everybody thinks they can have a go at it nowadays"

He suggested that when he retired at the end of the year; he could still have a financial stake in the business and would help us to try and find suitable properties to work on.

So, Debbie, her dad and me all agreed to give it a try and when I went into work on the Monday, I told Simon I was going to leave and gave him a months' notice. He seemed surprised but wished me all the best and later on in the day, Fred said to me, "Good for you John... you go for it"

A couple of years before all of this, Simon had hired this guy called Bob MacDonald, who I'm guessing must have been in his late fifties at the time. His job role was to be deputy production manager and Simon stressed to me that I would still be senior production manager. To be honest, I couldn't have given a toss because all those job title descriptions do nothing for me and I always remember looking out the upstairs tea room window one day, to see Simon with an aerosol can of white paint, spraying the letters DIR in three separate places. I knew exactly what he meant and it was an abbreviation of the word DIRECTOR and the three places were for himself, Fred and Matthew.

"Alright Si," I said when he came back upstairs, still holding the can, "Dir (pronounced der)... what's dir?" I asked.

"I beg your pardon?" he replied.

"You've wrote dir all over the floor outside"

"It's not dir... it's director!" he said looking all flustered and marched off to his office.

"Looks like dir from where I'm standing," I said to no one in particular and sparked up a cigarette.

So, Bob MacDonald started and when I first met him, he seemed ultra confident, which led me to think to myself, "Shit... he's gonna end up making me look naff," but it soon became clear that it was all for show and I needn't have worried.

I'm not saying he wasn't any good but rather less professional than he initially appeared to be and when it came to driving the forklift, he'd regularly drop pallets, which ended up damaging most of the paste tables. We ended up getting on really well which seemed to upset Simon and it didn't help that Bob spoke his mind and didn't care who he upset. I felt a bit rotten when it came to the time I was leaving because we'd become friends but Bob said he didn't blame me and wished me all the best, as did most of the workers on the shop floor. One of these workers called James was particularly upset about my moving on and along with Bob, as well as John, Jackie and Tony (from the office) he came for a drink at a nearby pub to send me off.

James was a funny old thing (actually not that old, he must have been in his mid-twenties) and to me, he was this Walter Mitty type character that lived in a fantasy world. He would tell me about all the women he had slept with and I always remember him telling me once that he 'had a Dutch bird on the go'

It was all total bullshit of course and in reality, he probably spoke to some Dutch woman for about five minutes or even less… but was it bullshit? I might be completely wrong and he could in fact have been the biggest stud in Harlow, but somehow, I doubt it.

Leslie (one of the Bethnal Green guys who had helped me with the gypsy kid) was also upset about me going too. As I've explained earlier, he had mild learning difficulties (cheap labour) but when it came to loading the trailers with paste tables and step ladders, there was no-one who could touch him. I don't mean he physically loaded the trailers (well, not too much anyhow) but rather working out how many we could get on them to maximise profits. Thinking about it now, I reckon he had some form of autism because he was absolutely brilliant with numbers, but that was something that didn't even enter my head at the time.

As of 2009, I now work as a woodwork instructor at a day service for adults with learning difficulties and I can honestly say that it's not only the first job I've ever liked, but loved too.

Anyway, back before I started that job, I always considered people with L.D as being 'a bit simple' (it sounds terrible now) but Leslie also suffered with epilepsy, which quite a few of the guys at the day service do too. Of course, we are trained in dealing with these situations but it makes me cringe now to remember Fred kicking Leslie (albeit softly) and telling him to "Get up and carry-on working" when he was having a seizure on the floor. How things can change in someone's life and although I'd always considered myself to be reasonably caring towards others, I am so much more now and am almost like another person.

I can remember telling Beige that I was leaving the company and him staring down at the ground and saying in a gentle voice, "Goodbye John…. I will miss you"

That was my last real memory of Beige and when I went to visit Simon about six years later, he told me that not only had Bob died of cancer, but Beige threw himself under a train and killed himself.

I couldn't believe it and was completely shocked. I'd always had this hope that he would one day return to Barbados to retire, but he never made it and must have been so depressed during the remainder of his life.

CHAPTER 8

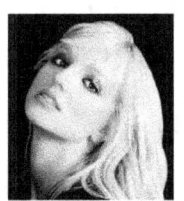

Predominantly, the main locations Ron (Debbie's dad) bought his houses from were in the Stratford, Leytonstone, Walthamstow, Leyton and Chingford areas and when me and Debbie first got together, he was in the process of having a brand-new block of flats built just off of Lee Bridge Road. I was nineteen at the time and we bought one of the top floor flats as an investment, with the idea of renting it out until we were ready to buy a house of our own and use the profit from the flat as a down payment. Me and Debbie got engaged the following year and Ron had just bought an end of terrace house in Chingford, with a plot of land on the side which he planned to build a new house on. We decided to buy the house he was doing up and once the new home was finished, we'd sell the house we were living in for a profit and move into the new home next door. Unfortunately for Ron, the agreed decision for him to build a new house on the land was overturned and the only option he was left with was to sell it to us. So, after getting married and living in our house for a couple of years, we decided to have an extension (which had been approved) on the land next door and it nearly doubled the size of the house. Being used to

BIPOLAR…..MAYBE?
(Volume Two)

driving forklifts, we hired a digger and I dug out the footings before they were filled in with concrete and the brickwork could begin. Just working on our extension gave me a lot of experience and Ron was great because he helped out a hell of a lot too.

By the time I started to work for Ron, me, Debbie and the kids had moved three miles up the road and had another extension on our new home. After that, I swore I would never do another because it is so disruptive, unless you can afford to move into a rented place while the work is being carried out, which was something we couldn't do. The plans for this extension (which had also been approved) required the footings to be dug to a depth of one metre and once again, I hired a digger to do the work. Once complete, I rang the building regulation guy to come and sign that part of the work off and he seemed satisfied the depth was correct. Satisfied that is until he saw what was a tiny tree about eighteen inches high, a couple of feet away from the front of the footings.
"I don't like the look of that tree," he said, "take a cutting to the town Hall in Ilford and they will be able to tell you what it is"
"And then what?" I asked.
"And then you ring me and tell me what they said"
I hadn't even noticed this tree (which seems an exaggerated description because it was so fucking small) but did what he said and cut one of the branches off, which was no thicker than a twig with a single leaf on it and drove to the town hall. I felt like a right idiot walking down a packed Ilford high street carrying this

PART ONE: TOIL

bleedin' twig and when I got to the town hall, I found the room dedicated to all things relating to trees and placed the twig on the counter before ringing the bell for assistance.

"How can I help you sir?" asked this tubby gentleman as he wobbled over while tucking into a sticky bun.

"Can you tell me what type of tree this is please," I replied.

"Well... there's not much of it but let me have a look in the catalogue," he mumbled whilst shoving the last bit of bun into his greedy gob.

He bent down under the counter and after much huffing and puffing, pulled out this thick brown book which he slammed down on the surface before us. He then got a tape measure and started calculating the size of the veins in the leaf before opening the book about halfway into it.

"Now let me see," he said and with two chubby fingers running down two separate lines of numbers that ran horizontally and vertically until they reached a point where his fingers met, he said out loud, "Page 97," and then flicked the pages until he reached that desired number. I didn't have a clue what he was doing and what all those numbers were that he was looking at.

"Ah yes, here we are.... Common Ash," he finally said.

"Common.... that's good isn't it?" I asked.

"That depends on the meaning of your description," he replied.

"Well... being common must mean there are a lot of them"

"This is true," he nodded.

"So does that mean they are less likely to be a problem

when situated two feet away from an extension we are undertaking?"
"Just the opposite I'm afraid… the Common Ash has a strong and wide root system and if two are growing together, they have to be at least sixty feet apart to ensure enough space for the development of each of their own root patterns, or else each tree could effectively strangle the other one to death"
"So it doesn't bode well for our extension?"
"No unfortunately, I'm sorry to be the bearer of bad news"
"Oh well… thanks for your help and now I have to ring the building regulation guy when I get home"
"Good luck"
"Thank you and goodbye"

"Hello," came the voice on the other end of the phone when I got back.
"Er hello, it's Mr. Barrett here"
"Hello Mr. Barrett…. did you have any luck finding out the species of our little tree?"
I could tell he was taking the piss but remained polite because when it came to progressing with our extension, he was god.
"Yes… it's a Common Ash," I replied with my fingers crossed.
"Hmmmm," came the response over the phone.
"Please be okay," I thought to myself.
"I will require the footings to be an additional one metre in depth"
"Fuck it!" I whispered under my breath.
"Pardon?"

PART ONE: TOIL

"I said, thank you. I'll get onto it straight away"
This was on a Thursday morning and I'd already told Simon (who I was still working for at the time) that I'd be in a couple of hours late that morning, but now I had to ring him again and say that I wouldn't be back at work until the following Monday. The main problem I had was that the majority of the footings were only two feet away from our next door neighbour's fence and because I'd had to start using the digger at the rear of the house and work my way to the front, there was no way I could use it again to dig the additional metre. The only option I had was to dig the rest by hand and at fifty two feet in length, I figured four days should give me just enough time to get the job done before the guys with the ready mix cement were due to come and fill it up. I could tell Simon wasn't too happy about it but what could I do? I had to get it done by Monday and so didn't have any choice. After speaking to him, I hung up, grabbed a bucket and shovel, jumped down in the trench and started to dig. It wasn't too bad at first but the deeper I got, the higher I had to swing the shovel loaded up with clay, into the bucket which was stood at the top of the footings. Two metres is just over six-foot-six and I'm five foot ten, so I'd have to go on tip toe when I got near to the required depth and on numerous occasions, the shovel would hit the side of the bucket and pull it down into trench. I would then have to grab the bucket, climb up a ladder and reposition it before climbing back down and starting over again. Ron kindly agreed to help but there was no way I was gonna let him do the digging because it was a real poxy job, but just by him taking the full bucket to the skip was

going to make a massive difference. Unfortunately, he couldn't get there until the afternoon and so I had to keep climbing up the ladder every time the bucket was full. It didn't help for two reasons that the weather was baking hot, the first because the heat was a killer but more importantly, as the clay begun to dry in the heat, large cracks appeared down the sides of the trench. This meant that as soon as I'd reached two metres deep and about six feet in length, I would have to shore up the walls of the footings with sheets of plywood, held to each side with lengths of four by two timber. I was knackered by the end of the Thursday but was up by six the following morning and stuck back down in that fucking trench again. Simon came round on the Saturday and gave me a hand, for which I was really grateful but I knew his main reason for doing so was because he wanted to make sure I was back at work on the coming Monday. In all, we filled eighteen skips with earth and clay and if the footings had only been one metre deep, then we could have halved that amount. It poured down with rain on the Saturday night which meant I was faced with ten inches of water on Sunday morning, sitting on the bottom of the trench. By now I was getting really pissed off with the whole thing but by early evening on that Sunday it was finished, but just after I climbed out the footings for the last time, a large section of the front corner caved in on itself, snapping the four by two timbers like twigs. It would have crushed me to death for sure had I still been in there but on the plus side; the building regulation bloke had paid a visit about an hour earlier and told me he was satisfied with the depth. Our house (in the middle of our street)

PART ONE: TOIL

sorry about that... the house was built in the early thirties and the original footings were only twelve inches deep. This meant the new footings had to go underneath the concrete so when they were filled, it would act as a key and help to create a more stable base for the extension. Because of the shallow depth of the old footings and the fact the new ones were starting to crack along their clay walls, we had to place 'needles' at strategic points along the outer wall of the house because there was a real risk our home might collapse due to the close proximity of the two metre deep trench I had dug. These needles were basically steel girders that passed through one-foot square holes on the outer wall and they were held up by Acro props at each end. There were five needles in total and once inside the house, they passed across the staircase which made it really difficult for us to get Nin upstairs because she was only a baby at the time and had only been born a few months earlier. I would have to struggle up the stairs first and then Debbie would pass Nin to me by weaving her in and out of the steels. Thank fuck it was only like that for three days, and twenty-four hours after the footings had been filled, we were able to remove them for good. The original bathroom was at the back of the house but we were going to convert it into an en-suite for our bedroom and had to remove most of the rear wall in order to position a twelve-foot-long steel across part of the original build, to the outer wall of the extension. The reason for this was part of the new bedrooms upstairs were cantilevered so they protruded over the ground floor extension, allowing us to have a side entrance to the garden and yet still obtaining

BIPOLAR.....MAYBE?
(Volume Two)

maximum width on the first floor. I had to screw the bathroom door shut for a couple of days because it was possible to go inside and walk off the back of the house if you weren't careful.

So back to the footings and imagine my relief when I was back at work on Monday and Ron rang me to say they had now been filled with cement, because the last thing I wanted to do was get back in that trench and remove the clay that had collapsed into it. Although that corner wasn't quite two metres in depth anymore, it was plenty deep enough and covered an area of over four feet square. You could have built a fucking tower block on it, I tell ya!

It was whilst I was down in the dreaded trench digging it deeper, that a shadow fell over me and when I looked up and squinted against the sun; I saw the silhouette of a man standing above me. I placed my hand just above my eyes in order to block out the glare and recognised him as this guy who stood in the porch of the house opposite to us, while he smoked a cigarette and I was filling a skip with clay from that fucking trench. We had nodded and waved at each other from time to time and I just assumed he owned the house but was surprised when I heard him start to speak.

"Gee… that's some project you've got going here," he said in an American accent.

"Just a bit," I replied before asking, "Have you just moved into the area?"

"Who me? No, no…. I just rent out one of the rooms when I come over"

"From America?"

"Is it that obvious?" he laughed.

PART ONE: TOIL

"Well…. I suppose you could be Canadian"
"That's a different accent entirely"
"Is it?" I said while climbing out of the trench and shaking his hand.
"John," I said.
"Hey John… I'm Ross, nice to meet you!"
"Likewise"
"That's a nice back yard you've got there," he said while looking over my shoulder"
"Yes, it is quite a nice <u>garden</u>," I replied.
"Okay, okay… I got it… garden"
"Only joking mate, I don't care what you call it," I said.
"I saw the people who lived here before you," explained Ross.
"Oh yeh… what were they like?"
"I only really saw the husband… a nigger"
I had to cringe because I absolutely hate that word but let him continue.
"While I was having a smoke on the porch, he would come out the house, open the passenger door to his car and then go back inside"
"What for?" I asked.
"I'm 99.9% sure he was a dealer because every time he'd do this, a car would pull up outside shortly after and the guy would come out of the house again and get inside this other car"
"Yeh… that would make sense," I said.
"Damn right 'cos it meant no phone calls, so no one listening in and it kept it away from his wife and kids"
"Don't you think they knew about it then?"
"Well she may have done but the kids were only small so I'm guessing he kept it from them"

"You should have gone over and got some from him," I said jokingly.

"I've already got my man for that and the stuff he supplies is swee-ee-eeet!"

I really had to get on with digging the footings and apologised to Ross that I had to carry on with the work.

"That's fine John... perhaps we could go for a drink in the Cricketers some time?"

The Cricketers was the nearest pub to us and was just up at the top of the road.

"Yeh... that would be great," I replied while climbing back down into the trench, "see you later mate"

"Ciao!" he replied as he sauntered back across the road with his hands buried deep in his pockets (but not as deep as that fucking trench!)

PART ONE: TOIL

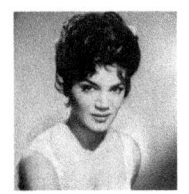

CHAPTER 9

Sorry about that, I've gone right round the houses (with extensions)... anyway, getting back to starting work for Ron. The main guy who did most of the work on Ron's properties was a man called Gary who had also worked on both our extensions, which meant I already knew him. He could turn his hand to absolutely anything and did it very, very well and taught me so much over the course of time. There was another guy who worked for Ron called Paul (who I mention in Bipolar.....Me?) and he did most of the house clearance and garden work, including putting up new fencing. It soon became clear that me and Paul had similar taste in music and he introduced me to an album by Eric Burdon called 'My Secret Life'

It's a fucking awesome record with no two songs on it the same and is one of those albums you can listen to, over and over again. Paul had a German Sheppard called Sonny who was so gentle and affectionate and I loved him to bits and would give him a great big hug like he was a teddy bear. I'd always loved German Sheppard's since I was a kid when my mum and dad lived in Chigwell and I used to sit by the window for ages, looking at an Alsatian that lived in the house opposite and would stare back at me. It almost became like a habit and at certain points during the day, we would both sit by our windows. I'd beg my mum if I could have one as a pet but she always said no and as the years went by, that longing slowly began to fade… that was until I met Sonny, but by then I was with Debbie and just felt like we wouldn't have enough time to give towards it. The main reason for this was that Debbie ran an ironing service and was constantly working and when I'd get home and finished eating, I would then go out on the deliveries.

The first house I worked on was in Walthamstow and whilst Paul and Sonny were out in the garden, I was in the back bedroom stripping wallpaper off the ceiling. Because I was stood on a step ladder and the angle I was at, Sonny could see me from outside and when I looked at him, he came into the house, up the stairs and laid down next to me at the bottom of the steps. It was as if he knew I was alone and wanted to keep me company and that blew me away. Paul was one of those blokes who it would take time for him to warm to somebody (if at all) but we seemed to click straight away and I think him finding out I was a fan of The Doors helped in no small measure.
To earn some extra money, Debbie started buying tickets for gigs and would then hold onto them until only a few days before the artist was due to perform, before selling them for a profit on eBay. She did pretty well for the first couple of months but, like anything, more and more people started doing the same thing until the profits became smaller and smaller until it just

PART ONE: TOIL

wasn't worth doing anymore. When she finally stopped in this venture, Debbie still had a couple of tickets left for a Santana gig at Wembley Arena and she suggested I go along with Paul to see the show. To many people this would have been a pretty small gesture but Paul was really grateful and couldn't thank me enough (even though it was Debbie's idea) and we ended up becoming very good friends.

I remember working on a terraced house in Chingford with Gary and Paul and in order to increase the size of the kitchen so we could get units on either side, we had to take down the wall adjoining the dining room and build a new one to make the kitchen about two-feet wider. However, doing this made the dining room smaller and so to compensate, we then removed the chimney stack so the room could be big enough to fit a dining table and chairs. This turned out to be standard practice for nearly all of the London houses we worked on (most of their kitchens just weren't big enough) and taking down the chimney stacks never seemed to be much of a big deal. That is until we started attacking this one with sledgehammers and the fucking thing just wouldn't budge… it was bleedin' indestructible!

We ended up having to hire a Kango (concrete hammer drill) to take the thing down, but even then, it took hours and hours and to be on the safe side, we held a long plank up against the ceiling with two Acros. Eventually we took a tea-break when the chimney stack was about two-thirds removed and suddenly there was a banging on the front door. Upon opening it, I was faced with an extremely angry looking woman who I recognised as being the neighbour and she told me to follow her into

BIPOLAR…..MAYBE?
(Volume Two)

the living room of her house. I wasn't sure why but I complied nonetheless and upon entering the room, I was confronted with smashed figurines and pictures hanging from the walls at funny angles. I say funny but this woman certainly wasn't amused and she began yelling at me, "I've been knocking on your door for the last twenty minutes but you purposely ignored me!"

Trying (badly) to calm her down, I replied in a soothing tone, "I'm terribly sorry but I didn't hear you"

"Of course you never fucking heard me, you had that fucking thing blasting and banging away in there!"

"I'm sorry, I…"

"I thought the fucking house was gonna come down around me!" she yelled while picking up pieces of her figurines and gently placing the broken bits on her coffee table.

"That was an heirloom from my late mother," she mumbled and tears began to form in her eyes.

I felt bleedin' terrible and promised her we wouldn't use the Kango anymore, but explained it would take longer to remove the chimney stack without it.

"I'm going out for an hour," she explained while taking down her crooked pictures and putting them on the floor, "you can use that thing but just make sure you're finished by the time I get back!"

I finally managed to return next door and explained the situation to Gary and Paul and we stared out of the front window to see her leave, before starting with the Kango again.

Thankfully we managed to get the chimney stack completely removed before she got back and looking at our watches, we realised it was nearly home time.

PART ONE: TOIL

"I know what I can do to cheer her up," said Gary, and with that, he placed a ladder up against the front of her house and filled in a crack in the rendering above the upstairs window.

Pleased with his work, Gary put the ladder back on top of his van and we all said our goodbyes before heading off home.

The next morning when arriving at the house and thinking no more about the previous evening, I was confronted with the woman standing outside her house with her arms crossed and a very angry expression on her face.

"Look what you've done to my house!" she yelled while pointing up at the filled crack above her window. Not understanding why she was angry, all I could say was, "I thought you'd be pleased… we filled the crack in for you"

"Pleased? Fucking pleased! That crack wasn't even there before you started that fucking racket!"

"Ah," was all I could answer.

"I'm going to work now!" she shouted, "Just make sure it's painted over before I get home and if it's not, I'm calling the fucking police!" and with that she got in her car, slammed the door shut and wheel spinned away.

"That's a great start to the day," I told myself and went inside to put the kettle on.

An hour later, an eighteen-foot steel girder arrived and me Gary and Paul struggled for the rest of the day to get in into position where the chimney stack had been, up in the ceiling.

"I'd better paint over that crack now before she gets home said Gary, and went outside.

BIPOLAR…..MAYBE?
(Volume Two)

It took about another three weeks to get the house fully finished before moving onto the following property, and I promised myself we wouldn't have any issues with the neighbours this time round… yeh… right!

PART ONE: TOIL

CHAPTER 10

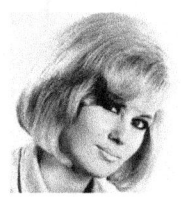

The next house we worked on turned out to be my first bungalow and it was in this lovely little village called Pilgrim's Hatch in a residential suburb of Brentwood, Essex. The bungalow was a semi-detached house and one of eight situated at the end of a cul-de-sac, which shared a driveway with a house on its right. Me and Debbie had actually found this one ourselves, without her dad's help for the first time and it didn't appear to need any real major alterations before we were ready to sell it.

By this time, Debbie's mum and dad were looking to downsize and Ron liked the bungalow so much and seeing its potential, he persuaded Debbie's mum that they could move into it when it was finished. This was all well and good apart from a couple of problems; the first being our profit margin would suffer and secondly, Ron was coming up with more and more ideas on how he wanted the bungalow finished. Of course, we didn't mind doing the extra work, Ron was going to pay for the additional costs anyway, but it did mean us spending more and more time on the property, which in turn meant it would take longer for us to move onto the next house.

BIPOLAR…..MAYBE?
(Volume Two)

So, we'd been working on the bungalow for a couple of weeks and during tea-break one day, we were sat on the patio and I looked over to the shared driveway and noticed a frog hopping away from the neighbour's garden gate. It was one of those cast iron gates you could see through and as a result, I knew they had a pond in their back garden. Worrying that the frog was going to hop down towards the end of the drive and get run over, I dutifully picked it up and pushing my arms through the bars of the gate, threw the little fellow back into the pond. Thinking no more about it but happy with my good deed for the day, I returned to my cup of tea and was about to light up a cigarette. Just then, the neighbour came out of her back door and started ranting and raving about something or other. Having no idea what the bleedin' hell she was going on about, I walked over to the gate and asked her to repeat herself.

"A snake just had that frog in its mouth!" she explained, looking rather flustered.

"Eh?"

"A grass snake… it had the frog in its mouth but he managed to escape"

"That's good," I replied, not knowing what else to say.

"It's not good you fool; you've just thrown the frog back into the pond!"

"So?"

"That's where the snake is!"

Upon hearing this, I looked at my hand and noticed it was covered in blood.

"Oh shit," I mumbled and realised I'd probably signed the frog's own death warrant, "I didn't realise… sorry about that love"

PART ONE: TOIL

"Why don't you just mind your own business and leave things alone?"
"I thought I was helping the frog out"
"What... by throwing him back to the mercy of the snake? You bloody idiot... and don't call me love!" she yelled, then returned to her house and slammed the door shut.
"That's the last time I'm getting involved with the fucking neighbours," I told Gary and sparked up my cigarette.

Several days later, Ron came round and had more and more ideas about how he wanted to improve the garden. This included the taking down of a really tall fir tree that stood next to the fence of our adjoining neighbours (on the other side) which I thought was a shame because it added to the overall charm of the garden. He said he would organise the tree fellers (I suppose it could have been women too) and asked me to inform the neighbours whom the tree was next to.
"Marvellous!" I thought to myself, but this time I was determined to handle the situation properly and after all, what could go wrong? I'm informing them in advance of our intentions so surely, they should be grateful.
"Good luck," said Gary with a grin on his face and off I went, feeling pretty confident the neighbour would appreciative of my news.
Things didn't bode well from the outset because as I walked up to the front door, I could hear raised voices coming from the other side. Well... when I say voices, a single voice would be a more accurate description and

BIPOLAR…..MAYBE?
(Volume Two)

I assumed (correctly as it turned out) that the wife wore the trousers in the relationship and the husband was this meek and mild individual with no say in things (the poor sod)

I was very tempted to turn around and come back at a later time (much later) but decided to bite the bullet and knocked on the door. All went quiet from inside before I heard the woman say, "Who's that?!" and then the sound of foot steps coming in my direction.

"Yes?!" she asked as the door flew open and I could see she was bright red in the face.

"Erm… I'm from next door and…"

"I know who you are!"

"Oh, er… well, it's like this…"

"I hope you've come to apologise for the noise!"

"Er, well no… I mean yes but there's something…"

"Come on, come on… I haven't got all day!"

"It's about the fir tree in the garden"

"Yes… what about it?!"

"We're going to take it down and I thought it best…"

"Take it down!"

"Yes and…"

"You can't take it down!"

"Erm… well we can and I've come to…"

"But you can't! It's… it's a nesting home for Pipistrelle bats! Pipistrelle bats! You've heard of bats, haven't you?!"

"Yes, but I'm sorry… it's still coming down"

"You fucking London lot are all the same. You come out here and think you can do what you like!"

I noticed in all this time that the husband was nowhere to be seen and I reckon he was hiding out the back.

PART ONE: TOIL

"I only came round to tell you, I didn't have to," I said and turned my back on her before walking away.

"Did you hear that?!" she yelled while shutting the door, "They're going to take the fir tree down!"

"What happened?" asked Gary as I walked back into the living room.

After explaining the situation, he thought for a while before replying, "That's bullshit, Pipistrelle bats nest in roof space, not trees"

"Do they?" I said, not having a clue.

"I know what she's trying to do," answered Gary, "Pipistrelle bats are protected and it's against the law to disturb their nests. She's trying to scare us into not taking the tree down"

Just then, there was a knock on the door and it was the same woman again.

"I'm warning you!" she yelled, "If you decide to go ahead and cut that tree down, I'll inform the police that you're breaking the law!"

"Those bats you're going on about don't live in trees," I replied, confident in my new learned knowledge, "so we won't be breaking any laws"

With that, she stormed off and two days later, the fir tree finally came down and I could hear her moaning in her garden all the while as the guys worked on it. I must admit, it was a real shame Ron wanted it removed because it was a lovely looking tree, but fortunately we didn't hear from the old bag again and we got out of that place as soon as possible. I never did tell Debbie's dad about the confrontation I had with her, because he might have changed his mind about moving in, but he never said anything about the neighbour, once he and

BIPOLAR…..MAYBE?
(Volume Two)

Debbie's mum started living there, so I'm guessing she must have calmed down and accepted the situation.

As I mentioned earlier, the buying and selling of houses only lasted a couple of years before my father-in-law's prediction came true and there just wasn't any money left in it anymore. Debbie asked me what I was going to do now and I really couldn't think of anything, but as she left the house one day to pick up some ironing, I told her I would look on the computer to see if I could find a job.
Debbie got home about ninety minutes later and immediately came straight into the office.
"Well… did you find anything?" she asked.
"Yes, two things actually," I replied, "There's a vacancy at a monastery to become a monk (do monks get paid?) or I could become a gigolo"
"What?!"
"A gigolo… but I've been looking into it and the only thing with that is I'd need to buy an Armani suit. You can get a half decent one for about a thousand quid"
"Don't you ever take anything seriously?" yelled Debbie and stormed out of the office.
In reality, I was really worried about being out of work and I was using my actions as a way of cheering myself up.
I let her calm down a bit before walking into the kitchen and apologised before saying, "Why don't I do some kitchen fitting or decking? I know how to do those things now"
I really didn't feel I was qualified to do much else but Debbie suggested I could do some tiling work as well.

PART ONE: TOIL

Just by sheer coincidence, on the following Monday morning when Debbie took Nin to school, she was talking to one of the other mums who explained that she'd just had some decking done and it looked absolutely awful.
"I told the workmen I wasn't paying for it," she said, "and asked them to take it away but they just left and I haven't seen them since"
Debbie said that I could do it again for her and that ended up becoming my first decking job, which included making some stairs leading down to the garden. Once it was finished, the husband and wife were really pleased with it and that gave me the confidence to continue, but if I'm honest, although decking looks good, I would never have it myself. It becomes really slippery when wet and constantly needs treating with decking stain every couple of years.
So, I started doing decking work throughout the summer and just by word of mouth, I found I had plenty of kitchen fitting jobs lined up for when the weather took a turn for the worse.
The following Spring, I was approached by a garden designer to do some decking at a house she was working on, and that led to a lot of work with her. My mate Paul who'd worked with me and Gary, benefitted from it too because the designer often wanted new fencing installed and that was his forte. When I think back on it now, I realise this woman was getting paid money for old rope because all she did was suggest what plants to buy and where to put them. You could have trained a monkey to do that but all of her customers were well pleased (mugs) and happily

BIPOLAR…..MAYBE?
(Volume Two)

handed over their hard-earned cash. Anyway, I wasn't complaining because I got plenty of work out of it and it was good to be working with Paul again.

Through contact with an electrician, I was introduced to a kitchen fitter called Pete, who was great at joining lengths of worktop together that ran at right angles to each other. Although there is a jig to perform this task with a router, I just couldn't get the hang of it and I ended up using Pete more and more, not just for kitchen fitting but other jobs too. It was almost like working on the houses we bought and sold earlier but the only difference this time was that we didn't own the homes. So, Pete would do the kitchen and plumbing too (which was handy) and I'd do things like tiling and decorating and when pricing each job, I took into consideration, Pete's cut as well. There was one particular house we were working on and the wife had just had a baby, so she spent as much time as possible at her mother's place during the day and told us to help ourselves to cups of tea. She left the house early one morning and after a couple of hours working, I told Pete that I'd make us both a nice cuppa. Upon walking into the kitchen and opening the fridge, I noticed a strange looking plastic bottle filled with liquid and quickly realised it was breast milk that the mum had expressed for the baby. I wondered what it must taste like but not willing to try it for myself, I poured some into Pete's cup and had some regular milk for myself. We both then went in the garden for a smoke and upon tasting his tea, Pete gave a funny look and said, "What's up with this tea? I bet it's that bloody skimmed milk… I can't stand it"

"Well, mine's all right," I replied and finally told him

PART ONE: TOIL

what he was drinking.
"You fucking bastard!" he yelled and so to make him feel better, I took a taste for myself and had to agree, it was bleedin' horrible.
Writing about that has reminded me of another occasion when we were still buying and selling houses. We'd bought a run down three-bedroom house and after installing the wiring etc, the whole place needed plastering because the walls and ceilings were in such a bad state. If there were only two or three walls needing doing, then Gary would plaster them but the whole house called for a team of men we knew and when they arrived one morning, I made them all a cup of tea and explained to the boss, who was called Richard, that we'd leave them to it and get out of their way and that I'd be back later in the afternoon. While we were talking, Richard's phone rang and his ring tone was that of an old woman yelling some obscenities. It really made me laugh but not as much as when he told me that he'd been to a baptism the previous Sunday and had forgotten to turn his mobile off. While everyone was sitting quietly in the church, his phone happened to ring and the silence of the building was filled with the screaming words, "ANSWER THE FUCKING PHONE YOU DOZY CUNT!"
Now that did make me laugh, and when I returned later that day, I couldn't believe they had finished the job in such a short amount of time.
So back to working for myself, with the occasional help from Pete, and I was lucky enough to find steady work although it was pretty difficult earning a decent profit out of it. This went on up until 2008 but my marriage

BIPOLAR…..MAYBE?
(Volume Two)

had definitely been in a rocky state for the last eighteen months because we still weren't earning enough to pay the mortgage and as I explained in Bipolar….. Me? I left Debbie in the September of that year. That's when things really began to spiral out of control and not knowing why, I was becoming really argumentative with the garden designer woman just because we disagreed on trivial things. In the end, she stopped using me (I couldn't blame her) and I was finally diagnosed with bipolar and sectioned a short time later.

PART ONE: TOIL

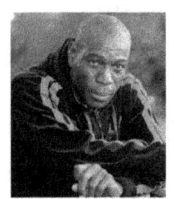

CHAPTER 11

Loughton School, 1980
Just like in every classroom, in every school in the world, there is the obligatory fat kid and ours was no exception, with a rotund lad going by the name of Martin Whale (he was as big as a fucking whale too!) It was during an English class one day, and we were all working hard (well, everyone else was except me) and out of sheer boredom, I got a ruler and decided to measure Martin's arse. He was sat in front of me, so I had to quietly slide my desk forward and then shuffle my chair along with it until I could lean forward and begin my careful measurements. So big was his monumental behind however, that it was only possible to measure one buttock at a time and even then, my ruler was only just big enough. Unbeknownst to me, not only had the teacher spotted me, but so had the rest of the class and they all stopped working to observe me undertaking my important research.
"Barrett... what are you doing?" called out Miss. Lloyd, with a curious expression on her face.
Her voice startled me because I was so wrapped up in what I was doing and leaning back into my chair again I replied, "Oh... er... nothing"

BIPOLAR.....MAYBE?
(Volume Two)

"He's measuring Martin's arse Miss," said Katie Finch, and with that, everyone burst out laughing (except for Martin that is)

"We say bottom in this classroom Katie... not arse," replied Miss. Lloyd, and the whole class started laughing again.

"No, I wasn't you liar!" I called out to Katie, while carefully placing my ruler back on the desk, and looking at Martin's angry expression when he turned round to face me.

"He was Miss, I've been watching him," replied Katie with a smirk on her ugly mug.

"Why were you watching me and not getting on with your work then?" I asked.

"Because I had already finished," came her smug response.

"More to the point Barrett," said Miss. Lloyd, "why weren't you getting on with your work?"

"I... er... I've finished too," I replied, which happened to be true.

We had been working on an essay explaining a traumatic incident in our lives and being someone who liked to write stories, not only had I finished mine (a serious piece regarding a recurring nightmare I'd experienced earlier in my childhood... oh yes, very high-brow) but I had written my friend Robert's too, who was sitting next to me. Miss. Lloyd was one of the kinder teachers at the school and after motioning for everyone to calm down, she gave the rest of the class ten more minutes to finish their stories before asking random pupils to read their work out loud. The first pupil she chose was Robert and I was beginning to

PART ONE: TOIL

regret helping him out.

Rob got to his feet, cleared his throat and then started to read his / my story.

"Once upon a time, I went to the shops to buy…"

"Has it got a title?" asked Miss. Lloyd.

"Oh, er… yeh," replied Robert.

"Yes"

"Eh?"

"It's yes… not yeh. This is an English lesson after all"

"Oh right, yeh… I mean yes"

"Well?"

"Well, what?"

"What is the title of your story?"

"It's er… it's called The Dirty Old Git"

Again, the whole classroom burst out laughing but Miss. Lloyd didn't look too happy and I was thinking to myself, "I knew I should have put 'man' instead of git"

I was hoping to add a little amusement to Miss. Lloyd's day when she finally got round to reading Rob's story, but had no idea she was going to ask him to read it out in front of everyone.

"Carry on," said Miss. Lloyd once the class had quietened down again.

"… to buy… to buy some sweets and once I had given the lady her money and waited for my change, I noticed a man standing right next to me with his hand on my arse… I mean bum"

More laughter ensued and I was glad my masterpiece was being well received.

"Change that to bottom before you hand it in," said Miss. Lloyd.

BIPOLAR.....MAYBE?
(Volume Two)

"Will everyone stop going on about arses and bums!" yelled Martin Whale before looking back down at his desk and falling silent again.

"Yeh!" called out my mate Chris, "He can't help it if he's got a massive one!"

By now the whole room was filled with laughter and it took a couple of minutes for Miss. Lloyd to regain calm amongst her pupils.

"Now Robert... carry on," she finally said, "and I'll have no more interruptions"

"Er... er, where was I?" mumbled Rob.

"Arse... I mean bum," said Chris and then immediately apologised so as not to get reprimanded.

"Bum," repeated Robert. "Once the lady gave me my change, I hurried out of the shop to make my way home but I noticed the man was following me and he was getting closer and closer"

By now, a hush had fallen over the classroom and I realised everyone was eager to find out what happened next.

"Suddenly," said Robert, "the man reached out and pinched one of my buttocks and..."

"Change that from buttocks to sweets," explained Miss. Lloyd, "Carry on"

"...and I ran even faster than before. It was no use however because the dirty old man caught up with me and gave the other buttock... er... sweet a pinch and then pulled down my tracksuit bottoms"

"Stop going on about bottoms!" yelled Martin again.

"He ain't talking about his arse... he means his trousers," I told him, before adding, "Carry on Rob"

"...pulled down my tracksuit bottoms and reached

PART ONE: TOIL

round to grab my test... test... test... what does that say John? I can't read your writing"

"Oh gawd!" I thought to myself, "He's given the game away.

Even though we still had ten minutes to go, Miss. Lloyd called out, "Class dismissed!" and as everyone shuffled out of the building, she said to me, "Not you Barrett, I want to speak to you... and bring your text book with you as well!"

So, after everyone else had left the room, she motioned for me to stand in front of her desk and told me to show her my own story (well... the other one was mine too but you know what I mean)

Silence filled the room for the next couple of minutes as she read my story, until she finally put it down and rested her hand on the page.

"I don't understand you John," she finally said in a softer tone, "here you have written a perfectly good story... okay it's not great but it's good, and if you paid more attention in class and stopped doing silly things like that story of Robert's, you could actually end up becoming a very good writer"

It was the first time a teacher had praised me like that (apart from a couple of times in art and technical drawing, even though my work was always grubby because I failed to wash my hands) and I promised Miss. Lloyd that I would try harder in the future... half meaning it too.

"I'm glad you have seen the error of your ways," she continued while drumming her fingers on my text book, "and I hope to see an improvement from now on"

"You will, I swear you will," I replied, "can I have my

book back now please? I'd better catch up with the others"

"Pardon? Oh yes, your book," she said and don't ask me why, but she turned the page over after my finished story and was faced with a drawing I had done of Martin Whale.

"It's idiotic behaviour like this which is exactly what I'm talking about!"

My eyes quickly glanced down at the drawing and I really had to struggle to stop myself laughing.

"I want you to go straight to the headmaster and show him exactly what you've been doing in my classroom!" yelled Miss. Lloyd and slammed the book shut before passing it back to me.

"But I'm going to be late for my science…"

"Headmaster! NOW!"

So, I was going to be late for my science lesson (at least something good came out of it) and made my way up to the main building where the headmaster was teaching maths to the year above mine. Now Harry (our nickname for him) was very old school (literally) and was really strict, so it went without saying that I wasn't looking forward to seeing him. I timidly knocked on the classroom door but of course he couldn't hear it, so I had to knock louder.

"Yes!" came this booming voice from the other side and I very slowly opened the door… anything to delay the inevitable onslaught of abuse that was guaranteed to come my way.

"It's you Barrett! What do you want?"

The school only had just over two hundred pupils, so the teachers knew almost everyone by name… well,

PART ONE: TOIL

they certainly knew mine anyway.

"Miss. Lloyd has told me to come and see you," I replied timidly and started to walk towards his desk, with all the older kids jeering at me.

"Quiet... the lot of you!" yelled Harry as I finally stood before him.

"Well, what is it?!" he barked.

"Miss. Lloyd said I have to show you my text book," I said and passed it across the desk.

"What for!"

"Erm... I think she wants you to look at the last page"

Looking slightly confused, Harry laid the book down in front of him and opened it to the final page of work (if you can call it that)

"What is this immature nonsense?!" he bellowed and lifted the book, before turning it around to face me.

I had no choice but to stare at the offending page and couldn't control myself any longer. I began to burst out laughing, so Harry banged the book down in front of me, stood up and rushed round the side of the desk, before grabbing my ear and walking me out of the classroom. As we left the room, I could hear cheers coming from the older kids and knew exactly what was coming.

Harry stopped briefly next to a cupboard and from it he removed a cane, then led me into the changing rooms and bent me over one of the benches.

"Perhaps this will knock some sense into you!" he yelled, "But somehow I doubt it!"

He then whacked my arse / bottom / buttocks and bum three times before standing me up and grabbing my ear again. Back to the classroom he led me and while

BIPOLAR…..MAYBE?
(Volume Two)

dragging me to his desk, Murray McKenzie (the school bully) pinched my already stinging arse and for the briefest of moments I thought, "This is just like the story I wrote for Robert.

Upon reaching his desk, Harry opened the book again, ripped out the offending page and then scrunched it up and threw it in his bin.

"Now get to your next class!" he yelled and tossed the text book straight at me.

As I made my way to the science lesson and even though my arse was burning like mad, I still had the image of Martin Whale in my head and couldn't stop laughing.

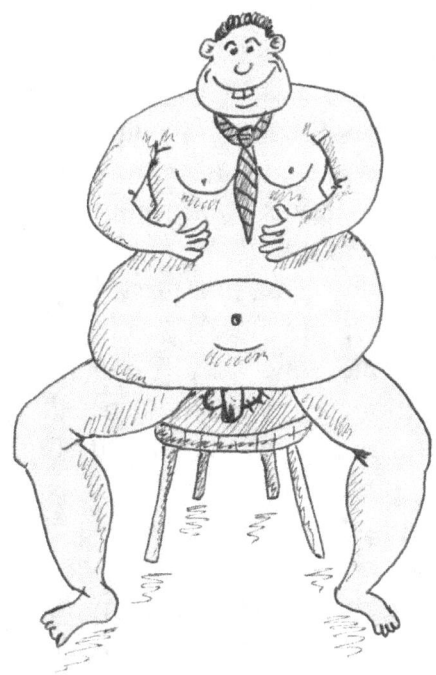

Not the original alas, but it's a very close interpretation

PART ONE: TOIL

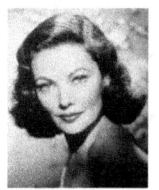

CHAPTER 12

It was on the following January and the full force of the wintertime had truly set in. Heavy snow had fallen overnight and because my mum and dad's house was situated about halfway down a pretty steep road, not only was my dad unable to get his car up the hill, which in turn meant he couldn't take me to school, but the train station I would usually walk to was closed and so I had the day off as a result... result! Most of my mates either lived a short distance from the school or the trains they would travel on were still running, and so they all made it in on that morning.

Throughout the day I made a great big snowman (it's got to be done... it's the law!) and in the afternoon the telephone rang and it was my friend Ed who had just got in from school. He explained that they had all got the cane for throwing snowballs (I thought that was a bit of a strict punishment) until he went on to say it turned into a big fight with the class above ours and quite a few kids got hurt.

Anyway, during the course of that night, it had stopped snowing and the gritting lorries were out in full-force up and down our road. The station had also been re-opened and so much to my disappointment, my mum

BIPOLAR…..MAYBE?
(Volume Two)

made me go into school and when I eventually got there, I discovered that all of my mates were pretending they couldn't make it in and so had the day off (They must have been jealous of me the previous day)

That afternoon, I started throwing snowballs at a group of girls from my class, when a prefect walked up to me and said, "Stop doing that Barrett, or I'll inform the headmaster"

What the fuck?! Who did this dickhead think he was? You can bet he became a copper when he got older and who was he, calling me by my last name?

"Fuck off Norris!" I told him, "Go and make yourself busy and tell someone else off for chewing gum"

"I'm warning you Barrett"

"Oh, piss off you wanker!" I replied and went to pick up some snow to throw at him but then had a much better idea.

There was a brick wall next to where I was standing and because it was old and everyone used to lean against it, some of the bricks had become loose and a few were lying on the ground.

"Who needs a snowball when I've got one of these?" I told myself, before picking up the brick and chucking it at the prefect.

Blimey, by the racket he was making, anyone would have thought I had hit him in the head instead of his leg, but he eventually quietened down and limped into the main building. Thinking no more about it, I decided to go for a smoke in our secret hiding place but before I had a chance to move, Harry the headmaster yelled from the building. "Barrett! Get in here now!" and I knew that fucking Norris had grassed me up.

PART ONE: TOIL

"Didn't you want to be left out… is that it?" he said while bending me over in the changing room.
"Sir?"
"Your friends… each of them received the cane yesterday!"
"Yeh, I know sir but it wasn't that…"
"Be quiet, I don't want to hear any of your excuses," he said and whacked me on the arse with the cane.

To be honest, I was expecting at least three but when no more followed, I felt pretty happy, even if my arse was stinging.

"Now get out of my sight… I don't want to see you for the rest of the day!" he said and pointed towards the door with the cane.

"But I've got you this afternoon for a maths lesson"
"Get out!"

So out I went and still had time for a cigarette before lunchbreak was over.

I can remember Martin 'Big Arse' Whale getting the cane once and just like something out of The Beano or Dandy, he stuck a book down his trousers and hoped that would absorb the force of the stick as it struck his ample buttocks. However, it was blatantly obvious to Harry because Martin's arse was now square and flat, and so once the book was removed, he got an extra caning for his efforts.

Very quickly and while I'm on the subject of snowballs, about a year later, I went to visit my mate Richard in Theydon Bois (we had moved away from the area when I was nine)

Again, it had been snowing heavily and we were on the

BIPOLAR…..MAYBE?
(Volume Two)

plain (the name we called a field next to the forest) having a snowball fight with two other kids we had never seen before. These two boys were about forty-feet away from us and unbeknownst to me, there was a man struggling to force a push-chair through the snow with a baby in it. One of the kids had just hit me on the side of my head with a snowball and I was determined to get him back, and so I scooped up a load of snow and formed it into a large ball before lobbing it at him. At that precise moment, everything seemed to slow down as I watched the snowball fly over the boy's head and hit the baby right in the middle of the face, causing the push-chair to topple backwards.

"Oh shit!" I said to Richard, who along with the two other kids, had watched the whole thing happen, and then I saw the man lifting the push-chair back onto its wheels and quickly checking the baby was okay before charging at me like a redrag to a bull (well… to be more precise, a bull to a red rag)

The two kids got out of his way and I just froze (in the freezing cold) to the spot as he got closer and closer, with the baby crying all the while behind him.

"It was an accident… I didn't mean it!" was all I managed to get out before he pinned me to the ground and began ramming my head up and down in the snow. "You fucking idiot!" he yelled with his face inches from mine, and with one final push, he got up and trudged his way back to his child.

I felt absolutely terrible because the last thing I'd wanted to do was hurt a baby, but by the time the father got back to him, he had stopped crying and so I'm guessing he must have been all right.

"Stupid bloke," said Richard, "What's he doing pushing that baby along in the snow for anyway?"
I just nodded my head silently and could feel my face blushing, not just with embarrassment but with shame also.

Anyway, back to the school and a few days later we had a drama lesson (what a waste of bleedin' time that was, but it beat doing maths)
The teacher who ran the class was called Mrs. Hooley and you could tell she was an ex-hippy with a real laid-back approach to teaching, with her skinny jeans tucked into a pair of multi-coloured socks and a pair of round, John Lennon type glasses. Our class was divided up into groups of six and each group had five minutes to perform a short play based on moments in history. Of course, I had to direct our group's effort (to me it was the film I would never make) and the group consisted of Martin Whale, the kid with the massive arse (did I mention he had a big arse?), Robert, Ed, Chris, Simon and me (multi-tasking... impressive eh) Except for Martin but along with Simon's girlfriend Susan, as well as Jerrod who was in the year below us, this turned out to be the same group of people who ended up going on holiday to Tenerife in 1986 (see volume one)
I had decided that our play should re-enact a part of the Battle of Hastings (not that I knew much about it) with a battalion of Normans attacking one of King Harold's castles. The reasoning behind my choice of subject was purely down to the fact that I wanted us to make use of the wooden gym equipment that was attached to one of the walls, and could be swung out on its hinges when in

use. This equipment included two ladder-like contraptions which were about twenty-feet in length and could be removed from the rest of gear and used as either monkey bars or climbing frames, but my idea was much simpler and I wanted them to use as ordinary ladders. The idea was that the main part of the climbing frame stayed attached to the wall and could act as the high battlements of the castle with two defenders (Chris and Ed) positioned at the top. The ladders were leant at a steep angle against the battlements and on the ground below, were a pair of blue crash-mats acting as part of the moat. While Martin and Simon stayed at the bottom of the ladders to oversee any technical problems (or scream for help if anything went wrong) me and Robert pretended to be two attacking Normans and climbed the ladders to try and breach the castle. As we neared the top, Chris and Ed threw lethal rocks (rubber balls) at Martin and Simon and finally pushed the ladders away so they went swinging down onto the crash-mats, with me and Rob still hanging on tightly. In order to stop ourselves from getting injured, we gripped the top rung of the ladder with outstretched arms that stayed completely straight, so it wouldn't hit us when we landed on the mats. So, our five-minute play consisted of four minutes getting the thing set up, thirty seconds of action and a final thirty seconds admiring the screaming adulation we received from the rest of the class (total silence)

"Very good!" said an enthusiastic Mrs. Hooley, who didn't in the slightest seem concerned about the dangers involved it took to create our masterpiece.

There's no way we would be allowed to do that

PART ONE: TOIL

nowadays but in the unlikely event that we were, you could bet we'd have to wear special harnesses and hardhats and safety goggles and all that malarky.

Seeing as the class was short of a few people that day, I asked Mrs. Hooley if my troupe of artistes (me and my mates) could perform another short play as a grande finale for the day's proceedings, to which she kindly agreed. Our moment in history was this time based on the terrible events of the 15th of April 1912, when the RMS Titanic sank on its maiden voyage. This was long before that crappy movie with Leonardo de Cappuccino and Kate what's her face (watch the 1958 film 'A Night to Remember' it's miles better… or should I say fathoms) and I was determined to be 100% respectful to the subject and treat it with dignity it deserved.

I had originally thought we'd only have enough time to perform one play and even though we had rehearsed two (because I couldn't make my mind up which one I liked the most) I thought the attack on the castle would be the most exciting of the two. Seeing how the audience response to that play had been a bit of a let down (to say the least) I was pleased we might have a second chance to redeem ourselves and win them over. The piece involved quite a bit of setting up, which we undertook while the play before us was performing, and involved Martin standing behind the gym balancing beam, which doubled as the bar of the main saloon on the ocean liner. We had four crash-mats in total and when rolled up, we used them as giant pillars which were supposed to be holding up the ceiling of the saloon. They must have been about three-feet in diameter and ten-feet tall and were heavy enough for

BIPOLAR…..MAYBE?
(Volume Two)

two people to struggle when trying to lift them.

So, Martin was the jovial barman and the rest of us were well-to-do first-class passengers, enjoying our brandies and cigars as the ship began to list.

All of a sudden, a yell came from one of the ship's stewards (Martin in an Oscar performing double role) telling all the passengers to come on deck, and for the women and children to start boarding the lifeboats. The saloon barman began to make his way out of the room, but was called back by the five sophisticated customers who demanded he serve them more beverages.

"But the ship's going down!" he yelled, trying to reason with them.

"There's no rush my good man," explained one of the posh gents (Chris with a totally unconvincing accent), "There's plenty of time before any drastic action must be undertaken"

"But…"

"Now pour us four more rather large brandies… there's a fine fellow"

"But the ship is…"

"And have one for yourself too"

"Ooh… thank you very much"

We then spent the next minute pretending to get pissed and started staggering all over the place.

"Is it me Rupert, or is the saloon tilting at a queer angle?" said Simon to Ed.

"You've had one too many brandies old boy, ha, ha, ha" Then, in piece of acting worthy of Sir Laurence Olivier's undivided attention, Martin slid his folded arms across the length of the bar and fell down to the ground at the other end. The rest of us then spent the

PART ONE: TOIL

next two minutes falling all over the place and pushing the rolled-up crash-mats on top of each other while laughing and singing merrily to ourselves. Finally, a deathly calm fell over the scene before Martin got to his feet and addressed the audience.

"Yes ladies and gentlemen," he bellowed in a baritone voice, "these were the fortunate few who perished before the icy waters of the North Atlantic could consume them. They were brave, proud men who gave no thought for their own lives when a fine cigar and a large warming brandy was the order of the day... their like shall never be seen again"

We all then got to our feet as Martin called out our names: "The role of Sir Rupert Cosgrove was performed by Paul 'Ed' Edwards, Lord Bartley Butterscotch was played by Simon Higgs, The Earl of Worcestershire Sauce was acted by Robert Field, The Duke of Marlborough Lights was performed by Chris Anderson, myself... Martin Whale played barman Billy McGee and finally, the role of The Third Duke of Hazardous Material was played by John Barrett.

Just as the previous play had received a silent response, so did this one, but I allowed Martin to continue anyway.

"The play was written by John Barrett, set design by John Barrett, choreography by John Barrett, stunt supervision was by John Barrett and last but not least, it was directed by... you guessed it (I never told him to say that bit)... John Barrett.

Pleased with my efforts but disconcerted by the unenthusiastic reaction of the audience, I took my bow and scarpered quickly before things turned ugly and could hear boos and jeers as I left the building and went for a fag. It's funny when I think back, but I realise now that even though I liked to do things such as writing those silly little plays, I didn't want any speaking parts in them. I suppose I lacked confidence when performing something I had made up in front of the rest of the class, even though I enjoyed playing the fool in front of everyone.

PART ONE: TOIL

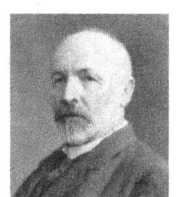

CHAPTER 13

Every pupil was given a kind of diary when first starting at the school, and the homework subjects were listed on each particular day (Monday to Friday) for the parents to sign, to prove the homework had physically been seen done. Of course, it goes without saying that I'd already learned how to forge my mum's signature and I don't think she ever saw that book in all the time I was at the school.

I liked Martin Whale a lot and just like the book he put down the seat of his trousers, another of his comic book style antics involved him spilling a whole bottle of ink over that week's pages of the homework diary, so the headmistress (Harry's wife who we called Mar) couldn't tell if it had been signed or not.

I'm guessing like most private schools; Loughton had its rituals for any new boys starting and all of us went through them at one time or another. The first (and least humiliating) was being pushed into a great big holly bush which stood next to Harry and Mar's private quarters. This was quickly followed by a trip to see the brown goldfish, where you would have your head pushed down a toilet before it was flushed, but only the unfortunate few got to see the actual brown fish. The third and most painful ritual was a date with the knacker racker tree, a gnarled and knotted tree stump that couldn't have been any thicker than a drain pipe. There would be four kids holding the victim by his arms and legs, and he'd be carried to the tree and positioned with the trunk in-between his legs before being pulled up and down it, resulting in a pair of bruised and battered bollocks. As I mentioned earlier, the school bully was this boy called Murray McKenzie and it was usually him and his mates who carried out the school-starter rituals. Although by no means tall, McKenzie was a stocky kid with a typical bully boy's mean face and a few years after leaving school, we saw him in a pub and whereas we had all grown taller, he was still this little short arse who we could have almost stepped on. He seemed all meek and mild, as if he were afraid we would beat him up at any moment, but none of us was that way inclined and left him alone. Like most new starters, I hated those rituals but my dislike for them was for a different reason than most. To me it was this private school crap that some of those pupils would continue into their adult lives and live by the old school tie code and carry on being dickheads forever.

By now, I'd been at Loughton school for nearly two years and on one summer's morning, a girl in my class called Andrea Spencer asked me if I wanted to go out with her. This came as a complete surprise to me because nearly every single boy thought she was the prettiest girl in the whole school, so of course I said yes. Gawd knows what she saw in me 'cos I was a right idiot who was always messing about and I can only assume

PART ONE: TOIL

the break-up she'd recently had with a boy in another form had done something to her head! This other boy was a cool, intelligent, sporting sort (a bit like The Kink's David Watts) whereas I was an uncool, unsporting and unacademic type, so maybe she wanted someone completely different… and she certainly got it. I was one of those boys who was always the last to be chosen for the hockey team (I hated sports and I don't care who knows it!) and I was put in goal every single time. My mate Robert was usually the second from last to be chosen and he was put in defence, which was fine by me because at least then I had someone to talk to. When a few of the other team's members came thundering towards us, Robert would mind out the way and I would cower behind the goal, so as not to be hit by the ball.

"Barrett, you fucking idiot!" came the response from my fellow team mates, but they soon left me alone and began attacking the other team's defence.

During these moments in the game, Me and Rob would pretend our hockey sticks were shotguns and we'd blast each other and fall dramatically onto the mud sodden ground. After the game had finished, we would all then have to march back to the changing rooms and take a freezing cold shower, no matter what time of the year it was (and people wondered why I hated sports)

A week before Andrea asked me out, a few of us went round to a friend's house after school on a Friday afternoon, still dressed in our school uniforms. His mum wasn't in and his dad was deployed in Northern Ireland as a bomb disposal expert, so we had the place

BIPOLAR.....MAYBE?
(Volume Two)

to ourselves. There were three boys, me, Chris and the kid whose parent's house it was (for the life of me I can't remember his name) and three girls... one of whom was Andrea. Chris had a pack of cards on him and suggested we play strip poker (I bet they were marked, the dirty git and he knew exactly what cards everyone had on them) This was all very well but none of us knew how to play poker so we changed it to strip snap instead, and we all sat round the dining table as Chris dealt the cards. Right from the outset, things didn't look good for me 'cos I lost the first go... then the second, the third and the fourth goes but luckily at that point my luck started to change. That was such a relief because I was just about to remove my trousers, but even better was the fact that Andrea started to lose the next few games and it was her turn to start taking some clothes off.

It got to the stage where she was only left wearing her skirt and bra and we were eager for her to lose again but alas; it was not to be. A few of the others lost a couple of times and had to remove a shoe here and a sock there and then it was my turn to start losing again. Off came my trousers and no sooner had I removed them, then Andrea picked them up and threw them out of the window. It was a three-storey house with the kitchen on the middle floor, which meant I had to run downstairs and out the front door in my undies, but luckily, no one else saw me apart from some old dear across the street. If it had been anyone else who'd thrown them out the window, I would have been really annoyed, but because it was Andrea... well, she couldn't do anything wrong in my eyes.

PART ONE: TOIL

So, she asked me out the following week and I can only put it down to the fact she saw me without my trousers on and could see just what a fine figure of a man I was (not!) Unfortunately, by the time I had returned to the kitchen, Andrea was fully dressed again and the game had come to an end. I needn't have worried though because in the coming months, I would get to see her undressed many more times.

On the odd occasions I didn't have to catch the train to school because my dad would drop me off on his way to work, I would usually be the first one there, along with Joy Wright, the clever kid in our class. She was a very well-spoken girl and would always let me copy her homework before the teachers turned up, which looking back on it now, was very good of her. Every Tuesday morning, we would have a home economics lesson, which could vary from wiring a plug to cooking a meal. On those occasions, we were required to bring a pint of milk in and I always thought how generous Barclays Bank in the high-street were for leaving me a bottle on their doorstep in the mornings.
Even though I disliked school enormously, I would still have days where I would be unexplainably happy and my mind would race all over the place. It was as if I were looking through the viewfinder of a video camera and everything was at high speed as though on fast forward and I was filming the grounds of the school with everything whizzing past me. It's really hard to explain and probably doesn't make any sense, but what confused me even more was that the very next day, I was filled with a deep melancholy and this time,

BIPOLAR…..MAYBE?
(Volume Two)

everything was in slow motion. Of course, I know what it was now but I just thought it was normal and everyone felt like that. Back in those days, it was described as manic-depression and the term bipolar disorder never even existed but if somebody had explained to me then that I was suffering from such a condition, I would have thought they were mad.

Me and Andrea were an item for about six months and thankfully in all that time, I was feeling really happy. It was great to see kids older than myself giving me jealous looks because every boy wanted to go out with her, but towards the end I kind of felt guilty for being in such a good mood for so long (bonkers I know) and decided to end our childhood relationship. It's funny but even now, I'm exactly the same and I am always the one to break up with a girl, because I know the pleasant sensation will increase at a very rapid pace until the highs become out of control and I end up doing really stupid things.

Every morning before school, me and my mates would meet up in an abandoned garage not far away and smoke cigarettes to our heart's content. We had rigged up a light bulb on a wire to an old car battery and even though nothing very much happened, we always felt like it was having our own place and it was great when the weather was pissing down outside. On this particular day, we had a double art lesson in the afternoon, which was fine by me because it was my favourite subject. After sitting down, we were each given a large piece of paper that must have been about three feet by two feet, and told by Mrs. Pearce the teacher, to paint a picture with its title being 'Street life'

PART ONE: TOIL

We could do anything we wanted just as long as it was relevant to the title and so in the very bottom right-hand corner, I painted a car parked next to a curb and on the pavement next to it was a scantily dressed woman leaning against a streetlamp. The man in the car was leaning across and saying something to her from out of the passenger window while she smoked a cigarette, with the smoke drifting lazily above her head. The light from the streetlamp cast just enough illumination to reveal this scene before it gradually grew dimmer and dimmer until 75% of the picture was in total darkness, save for several stars and the moon obscured by clouds. I was really pleased with the finished result but Mrs. Pearce took a totally different view and said that most of the picture was just "nothing"

"But it's a work of art," I replied, "I thought the whole idea was to express how we feel"

"And you feel an affinity with that man and woman?" she answered whilst staring at the image disdainfully.

"Well… no, but it's still a part of street life"

"Not where I come from it isn't," said Mrs. Pearce and moved on to the next desk.

I never did get to keep that picture and can only hazard a guess as to what happened to it. Probably stuck to the wall of the staff room so all the teachers could have a laugh and joke about it.

It was mid December and the weather was really mild for the time of year but it was pouring down with rain, so we started the day in the garage, fending off any other kids who wanted to seek shelter from the weather. Parent's evening was scheduled for that night and we were all pretty worried what our mums and dads would say regarding our work. I say mums and dads but I knew only my mum would be going because my dad never did, probably due to the fact that he could hardly read or write and he would have probably felt intimidated. While my mum was at the school, I spent most of the evening at home, worrying about what the teachers were saying about me. When she did finally get home, I ran upstairs to my bedroom but was immediately called down again and told to come into the kitchen.

"Er... how did it go?" I asked.

"Not too bad," she answered, "they all said you have the ability but need to try harder"

"Is that all," I replied, feeling relieved.

"Your English teacher said she is quite pleased with your progress"

"That's good"

"Even if you do have an overactive imagination"

I looked up at my mum and could see she had a smirk on her face and guessed the teacher must have shown her some of my work.

"And then I spoke to Mrs. Pearce"

"Ah," I said, remembering the Street Life picture I had done a few months earlier and was expecting my mum to talk about that.

"She said you all had to design a Christmas card..."

Shit, I'd forgotten all about that!

"Did she show it to you?" I asked.

My mum nodded her head and replied, "There are some things you just shouldn't do John, and that is definitely one of them"

PART ONE: TOIL

"Sorry mum," I said, "I realise that now"
The card in question depicted a snowy scene in a forest (nothing wrong there I hear you say) but that's about as far as the Christmas theme went. Parked askew upon the snow was an old Mercedes Benz with its driver door open and footprints leading away from it. The car was full of bullet holes and at the end of the trail of footprints, lay a blood-soaked man outstretched on the ground. A few feet away from the unfortunate man was a German guard holding a machine gun and next to him was Adolph Hitler giving a Nazi salute and shouting out, "Achtung! Merry Christmas!"
"What possessed you to do such a thing?" asked my mum and all I could do was shake my head in silence.
"Good job I didn't tell her about those comics you draw," she continued before patting me on the head and walking out of the room.

The oldest parts of Loughton school were purpose-built structures and began life as St. John's College before converting to Loughton School for Boys in 1889. Many of its former pupils were killed in both World Wars and there were three wooden plaques on the walls of the assembly hall, commemorating their names in gold lettering. Each morning in assembly, we would sing a couple of hymns and then pray for those departed pupils and although I'm not religious, I always felt it was the right and proper thing to do (even if I did make ill-judged Christmas cards from time to time) The main school building was situated at the top of an incline, with the assembly hall a little further down and then there were three more original classrooms at the bottom

BIPOLAR…..MAYBE?
(Volume Two)

of the hill. In-between the assembly hall and the three classrooms was the English room which sat adjacent to the playground, but this classroom was much newer and in reality, was nothing more than a glorified, giant porta-cabin rather than an actual building. The classroom where Harry laid scorn upon my 'work of art' was actually the main dining room and like much of the school, each room doubled for another which was probably due to a lack of space. Girls were allowed to attend the school from 1972 and when I started seven years later, I just accepted it for what it was and didn't know any different. My previous school had been an all-boy affair, which was okay but I much preferred there being both sexes at Loughton because some of the girls were really fit!

So apart from the girls and being someone who hated school, it goes without saying I would devise ways not to attend. I remember one particular time and I was genuinely ill (shock, horror!) and had been sick during the previous evening. Because of this, my mum let me take the next day off and as the hours passed, I was slowly beginning to feel better and better. Of course, it was great not feeling sick anymore but I somehow had to take another day off and set my alarm to ten minutes before my mum would usually get up. Racing down the stairs, I made my way into the kitchen and opening the lid to the biscuit barrel, stuck two Digestives in my gob and began chomping on them until all that was left was a ball of munched up biscuits. I then waited by the kitchen door and listened out for my mum to get up and as soon as she opened her bedroom door, I ran back to the fridge and took a large swig of milk. I then hurried

PART ONE: TOIL

to the downstairs loo and purposely leaving the door open, got on my knees with my head in the lavvy and started to swirl the milk and biscuit concoction in my mouth whilst making groaning sounds.

"Is that you John?" I heard my mum call out.

Moaning just loud enough for her to come to the door, I waited until she stood watching me and then… BBBRRRRRAAAAAAAAAAUUUUUUGGGGG!!!!

I'd moved my head just enough so she could get a better view as the Digestive/milk mixture came spurting forth and splattered the inside of the toilet bowl. I then looked up at my mum with a sorrowful expression on my face and some of the mixture dribbling from my mouth and down my chin.

"You can't go to school like that," said mum, "as soon as you stop being sick, go back upstairs to bed"

I nodded slowly and stuck my head back down inside the bowl again, with a few groaning noises added for good measure. I'd considered repeating the scam the following morning but thought it best not to because I didn't want to push my luck, and there was always the possibility my mum would wonder why my sick didn't smell like… well… sick.

Then there was the time I threw myself down the stairs but on this occasion, I waited until my mum was up and in the kitchen making herself some breakfast. Again, I was dressed in my uniform (to give the impression I couldn't wait to get to school) and standing on the top step, readied myself for the spectacle to come.

"Here goes," I said to myself and took a deep breath (I don't know why, it was only a short trip down the stairs) then dived forward, making sure to protect myself with

my outstretched arms as much as possible.
CRASH, BANG, WALLOP, "AAAARRRGGHH!!!"
It wasn't like Martin Balsam's character in 'Psycho' who almost runs backwards down the stairs while standing up, no... mine was a much more haphazard affair although probably more believable. Although that scene in 'Psycho' is technically brilliant, I can't help thinking that it looks a bit silly... I know, I know, I'm slagging off the master and I'm a fan of his too.
Lying spread-eagled at the foot of the stairs, I looked up to see my mum staring down at me with a concerned expression on her face.
"What happened?!" she asked frantically.
"I... I fell down the stairs," I moaned in response.
"What's going on?" said my dad standing at the top of the stairs with my brother next to him.
"He's fallen down the stairs"
A look of genuine concern appeared on my dad's face and finally he asked, "He ain't broken the bannisters, has he?"
He meant spindles but I knew what he was going on about.
"No, I haven't," I moaned, "I've damaged myself"
"Why... what's up with you then?" said my brother after descending the stairs and was stood next to my mum, staring down at me.
"I've hurt my leg"
"You look alright to me"
"How would you know? You're not a doctor!" I replied, hurt by his insinuation even though I was guilty.
"I was only..."
"Well don't!"

PART ONE: TOIL

As we were having this conversation, I was aware of my dad inspecting the spindles on the staircase for any sign of damage.

Davey then stared straight into my eyes with a look of suspicion on his face and I had to turn my head for fear of giving myself away.

By now my brother had left school and started going into work with my dad in the family business.

"Can you stand up?" asked my mum.

"I'll try," I replied and held my arms out in front of me, so my mum could help me get to my feet.

"That's alright mum, I'll do it," said Davey and I wondered what his game was.

So, he grabbed me by the wrists and started to pull but when I was about two feet off the ground, he suddenly stopped, even though he was still holding on to my arms. I had to think for a split second and then I realised what he was up to. Davey was hoping I would use my own strength to lift myself up the rest of the way, hence proving there was nothing wrong with me. I was left with no choice but to crash down to the ground again and then began shouting at my brother.

"What's happened?!" said mum.

"You bloody idiot, what did you let go for?!" I yelled and began groaning in pain again.

"Sorry mum I slipped," replied Davey, and I knew he was lying.

"Pick him up again," said my dad, finally happy the staircase was okay.

"I'm not letting him near me again… he's bleedin' dangerous," I said and could see my brother shaking his head slowly from side to side.

BIPOLAR…..MAYBE?
(Volume Two)

My dad then walked down the rest of the stairs, grabbed my wrists and pulled me up in a matter of seconds.

"Ooow… aaarhh, aaarhh… ooow," I moaned and finally, when upright, struggled to stand and told my mum I must have sprained my ankle.

"Go into the living room and lie on the sofa," she said and limping all the way, I was pleased with my acting performance and managed to get two days off school as a result.

Just as Davey was about to leave for work, he poked his head round the living room door and whispered, "You jammy git," and then he was gone.

I recently read in the paper about a kid who doctored his covid test to get out of going to school by sticking a strip of red paper on it where the positive line should go. Of course, his mum spotted it straight away but you've got to give him full marks for trying… that's my type of kid!

By 1989, Loughton School couldn't afford to stay open any longer, owing to the ever-decreasing number of pupils attending, but at least it made its first centenary. Even though I absolutely hated school, it was sad to know the place was finally demolished a few years later and the site was replaced with eight new houses. By coincidence, I happened to be doing some work on a house in 2008 with my mate Pete (the bloke who drank the breastmilk in his cuppa) and it backed onto the site where the school once stood. Even though there were no signs of any original buildings anymore, some of the trees had been kept from being chopped down and they now stood in the back gardens of these new homes.

PART TWO: RELAXATION

CHAPTER 14

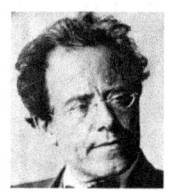

Spring 1982
All of the pupils at Loughton School received a letter to take home, regarding a trip to Italy and Austria during the half-term holidays. There had been other trips in my previous schools (although not abroad) but my mum and dad always said I couldn't go, so I thought there was no way they were going to agree to this trip (their reasoning was that they couldn't afford it, which was fair enough) Just as I thought, when I gave the letter to my mum, she read it and said no, but when I went into school the next day, all of my mates said they were going. I was absolutely gutted and later that night, I pleaded with my mum to ask dad, but knew what the answer would be. As she went into the living room to speak to him, I sat in the kitchen with my fingers (and everything else) crossed and waited for her to return. Eventually, my mum walked back into the kitchen shaking her head, but then began to smile and said I could go. I couldn't believe it and rushed into the living room to thank my dad.
"We can't do this all the time," he said without taking his eyes off the TV screen.
"I realise that dad, thank you," I replied and went back

PART TWO: RELAXATION

into the kitchen with a big smile on my face.

I really wanted to phone my friends and tell them, but I knew there was no way I'd be allowed (no mobile phones in those days) and didn't want to push my luck. It must be really difficult for the younger generation to imagine what it was like back then; no mobiles, no computers, no Facebook / YouTube / TikTok / Pinterest and the like, only one TV in the house with only three channels and until video recorders came in, that's all we were stuck with. The old saying goes, 'You don't miss what you've never had,' but not only did we not miss it, 'it' never existed in the first place.

I had to wait to go to school the next day to tell my friends (the only time I was looking forward to school) and our parents had to pay for the holiday in three instalments. So, the half-term holidays eventually arrived and the coach came to pick us up from the school entrance on a Monday morning and I thought how strange it was to see all these pupils in regular clothes and without their school uniforms on. Once all our luggage had been stowed away and we were seated comfortably, the coach set off for Luton Airport. I remember a group of us were quarrelling with some of the girls about which was the best music in the charts at the time, with the boys arguing for Madness, The Jam, XTC, Kraftwerk and the like, while the girls preferred George Benson, Kool and the Gang, ABC and all that stuff. Walkman's were really popular at the time and most of us brought our own to listen to on the journey, and I remember mine having two earphone sockets (very state of the art) so someone else could listen in too. The journey to the airport took about ninety minutes and once we could see airplanes taking off, we became really excited and knew we didn't have long to go.

In those days, smoking was permitted on planes and because me and my mates were lucky enough to be sat some distance away from any of the teachers, we spent the whole flight smoking away to our lung's content. Unfortunately, I can't remember where we stayed in Italy, I've tried looking it up but there doesn't seem to be a school record of it anywhere. I can recall the hotel being in a high street however, and was a bit run down, but that didn't bother us in the slightest. Five of us shared the hotel room; me, Ed, Robert, Simon and Chris and from the balcony, a kind of mini racetrack could be seen, with coin operated miniature cars running on electricity. One day, we were stood on the balcony smoking, and could see a boy in the year below us, steering his electric car through a gap in the tyres which surrounded the perimeter of the racetrack, and began driving along down the busy pavement. The owner of the racetrack was this big fat Italian man, and he was running along beside the car, smacking the back of this kid's head. We were all rolling about with laughter, especially when the car crashed into a table belonging to a café, sending the customer's cappuccinos smashing down to the ground.

The next morning, we took a trip to Venice, which entailed taking a coach to the nearest port before boarding a ferry to the ancient city. I remembered we visited the magnificent St. Mark's Basilica, this beautiful church that dated back to the 11th century and whose interior was even more breath-taking than the outside. My mates were bored witless but I was in my element and thinking about it now, that was probably the first time I began to appreciate such glorious examples of architecture. I can vividly recall my mood spiralling upwards as we walked around the church, taking in all the fascinating details, and the rest of the day's excursions only served to increase my mood.

"What's up with you?" asked Ed at one point, "You're acting all strange"

"I dunno," I replied, "I'm just loving every second of this place"

"Weirdo," he said under his breath and walked away to be with the rest of my friends as I lagged behind, savouring all the great buildings around me.

It fascinated me how instead of roads running through the city, there were canals and rivers and I couldn't get my head round how they built the houses and other structures in the first place. We walked along the many pavements, with each turn revealing even more splendid examples of architecture and I'm sure at one point I spotted in the distance, a small girl wearing a bright red coat disappearing around a corner! (I'm not telling you what it is, but you'd have to have seen the film to know what I'm going on about)

After a few days in Italy, we took a coach journey to a place called Zell am Ziller in Austria (I can only remember the name because I bought a plate for my mum with a picture of the town on it) and because it was out of the ski season, it resembled something out of Heidi in the summer months. Our hotel was a great looking building in a typical ski chalet fashion, and we were surrounded by mountains on every side. The town

BIPOLAR…..MAYBE?
(Volume Two)

itself was absolutely spotless and one day when my mate threw a sweet wrapper on the floor, this old lady told him off (gawd knows what she was saying) and made him throw the wrapper in the bin… if only people in this country cared as much. We were all allowed to spend some time without any teachers present, but were told to get back to the hotel at a certain hour. On one of these occasions, the five of us got absolutely pissed on an extremely strong local lager but luckily managed to get back to our room and into bed before a teacher poked his head round the corner to make sure we had returned. The next morning, I woke up pretty early and as my eyes were adjusting to the daylight, I thought I could make out a handprint on the wall next to my top bunk on the bunkbed. I wasn't too sure until my eyesight fully returned to normal and out of the window, I could see clouds where houses and shops had been the previous afternoon. Looking back at the handprint, I thought it resembled dried shit and my suspicions were confirmed when I took a deep breath and got a lungful of the foul-smelling odour which permeated every inch of the room. About six feet away from the handprint was another, then another and then they turned to footprints going across the floor, until they reached Ed's bed. He was still fast asleep and when I called out his name, he stirred and pulled the duvet around himself, revealing the white material to be completely covered in shit on the underside. By now, the rest of my mates had woken up and in unison they all called out, "What the fuck is that smell?"

This caused Ed to wake up but he didn't have a clue what happened during the night and all I could think about was him wandering round the room spreading his shit about while we all slept. We managed to sneak him into the bathroom across the hall without being spotted but there was no way we could dispose of the duvet and other bed linen, so we went downstairs for our breakfast as if nothing had happened. A short while later, the hotel manager approached Mr. Offord (our French teacher) who was sat at his table, and whispered something in his ear. I had to feel sorry for Ed because instead of coming to our table and asking quietly who did it, Mr. Offord stood up in the dining room in front of all the other kids and teachers and said in a loud voice while staring at us, "Who is responsible for defecating in their bed last night?"

We all looked at each other not understanding what he had just said, until he asked again but worded it differently this time.

"Who messed themselves last night?"

All the other kids burst out laughing and Ed finally put his hand up to acknowledge he was responsible. He didn't hear the last of it for the rest of the day, even though we took a visit to the beautiful city of Salzburg, with its amazing architecture and stunning scenery.

On the final day of our holiday, the teachers told us all to pack our suitcases after breakfast and then we took a cable car ride to the top of a nearby mountain, before walking along a winding track which led all the way down to the bottom. While almost still at the top and being the last in line of pupils, the five of us decided to take a short cut and make our own way back down before everyone else. Climbing over a fence that run alongside the track, we began to slowly navigate our way down an extremely steep hill, being as careful as we could, with one hand touching the ground to steady ourselves. It was no use however; such was the gradient and the slope caused us to stand up straight and then start running faster and faster down the hill. We had no control over our legs and the quicker we ran, the sooner we realised there was no way we could stop. In the distance but approaching at an increasingly rapid pace was another rickety old fence at the bottom of the hill and remembering the cable car journey, we realised that beyond the fence there was nothing… just a sheer drop of hundreds of feet. Our legs were now moving so fast, there was no way we could have gone that quick had we tried under normal circumstances and I called out to Robert that we had to trip ourselves up before it was too late. I don't know if you have ever attempted to do that but it is easier said than done, especially at the speed we were moving and I was the first to fall over before the others followed suit.

Over and over we rolled, over and over and over, with the fence getting nearer and nearer and it was a good job we tripped ourselves over when we did because we finally came to stop about six feet before reaching it. Our bruised and battered bodies remained motionless for about two minutes as we tried to catch our breath and when we finally stood up, we realised how lucky we had been. Looking along the length of the fence which ran horizontally across the bottom of the hill, I could see it eventually reached the track where the rest of the group were walking. Making our way to the track, we finally caught up with the others (who somehow hadn't even noticed we'd been missing) and

eventually made it down to the bottom of the mountain.
"What the devil has happened to you?" asked Mr. Offord when he finally had a chance to look at us.
"Er… we fell over sir," explained Simon.
"What… all of you?"
"Yes sir," said Chris, "we slipped on some grass"
All of us were completely covered in mud and grass stains and what made it worse was that we couldn't change our clothes because our cases had already been packed and were down in the reception area, along with everybody else's.
So, we had to get the coach to the airport and fly home covered in dried muck and I always remember my mum asking what had happened when the coach finally got back to the school and she was waiting for me. I told her exactly what did happen and all she said was, "You're lucky you didn't all kill yourselves, you silly sod," before driving me back home so I could have a shower and get into a fresh set of clothes.

In the December of that year, I turned sixteen and things began to change for the worse at school (if that were at all possible) and I decided that I would leave and join the family packaging business. That meant not taking any qualifications and much to my surprise, my mum and dad agreed. I think my dad didn't mind because he had no qualifications himself and always knew I would join the firm, and it was a great feeling when I finally ripped my school uniform to shreds, never to wear it again. Even though I didn't like the lessons, I was aware that the school didn't seem to have the same commitment when it came to educating its pupils, with many of the older teachers either retiring or moving on to teach in another school for the remaining few years of work they had left. A good example of the decline in teaching was during a geography lesson, where we were asked to draw a compass. By this stage, fewer and fewer pupils were joining the school and as a result, we merged with the other form in our year. Instead of drawing a geography compass with North, East, South and West being displayed, one of their boys drew a compass that you use to draw circles with. What made matters worse was that he was the head prefect for fuck's sake, but to be fair to him, it was a pretty good drawing. If my memory serves me well, that was the very last lesson I took and at the end of the school day, I didn't even look back when walking out of the gates.

CHAPTER 15

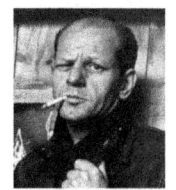

Theydon Bois, 1975
I'm guessing like most people; I can remember the first James Bond film I saw at the cinema, which happened to be 'The Man with the Golden Gun' in late December of the previous year and I thought it was absolutely brilliant. It was only years later that I realised it was one of the weaker Bond movies and my enthusiasm for it was probably fuelled by seeing it on the big screen. They say that the first actor you see playing Bond is your favourite and ITV showed 'Dr No' (the very first 007 film) in this year and in an instant, Sean Connery was the James Bond for me. Although I liked Roger Moore; Sean Connery seemed more dangerous and took the part seriously and my decision for preferring him was no doubt aided because my dad liked him the best (probably because he knew he was going bald like himself) even though he wore a syrup on screen. I know I'm a baldy too but I promise you that didn't influence my decision… anyway, I wasn't bald at the time 'cos I was only a little kid! It was because of ITV's screening of the Sean Connery Bond films (in the correct sequence) that I became a fan and loved every second

of them, and can always remember going to bed after each film had finished, imagining I was 007.

Even at a young age, I found that the Roger Moore Bond movies were becoming increasingly ridiculous and light hearted and by the time Pierce Brosnan's 007 came along, I gave up on them completely. It was only when the Daniel Craig version of 'Casino Royale' was shown on TV (I'd stopped seeing them at the cinema years earlier) that I realised the producers had gone back to the original formula, and reinstated Bond as the lethal killer he was originally intended to be. This 007 movie was easily the best I'd seen in years and because of it, Daniel Craig had quickly become my favourite actor to play the part. It was only after watching his subsequent Bond films, which were all pretty good (I haven't seen the last one and have really lost interest in seeing anymore) that I realised Sean Connery was still the best Bond by far. Although Daniel Craig plays the part very well and shows 007 to be the cold assassin he is, Sean Connery has everything the character should have. He is smooth and sophisticated but deadly and dangerous at the same time, shows just the right amount of humour without making the character seem ridiculous and has a way with the ladies that puts all the other Bonds to shame... even our Rog.

I'm probably in the minority but I also liked George Lazenby's solo effort, especially when he says at the beginning of 'On Her Majesty's Secret Service,' "This never happened to the other fellow" and Timothy Dalton was pretty good too. I just found Pierce Brosnan to be a bit of a pretty boy and a bit wooden (at least Roger Moore could raise an eyebrow when the right

PART TWO: RELAXATION

situation presented itself) Naaaah… give me Sean Connery any day of the week, even if he wasn't supposed to be a very nice person in real life. That honour goes to Roger Moore who would never forget his fans and would always give them the time of day when meeting them.

Sorry about that, I've really gone off on one there and the whole point I was trying to put across was that my dad had great taste when it came to films, and I loved watching them with him, whatever subject they may have been about. Like I've already mentioned, my dad could hardly read or write and I suppose to compensate, instead of books he would watch films, but the really strange thing is, every movie he liked was always highly rated by some of the best film critics in the world and that's why his favourite Bond movie (and mine too) is 'From Russia with Love' which is much more a spy film than the usual fare.

An early memory of mine was lying on my front on the floor, watching all these great movies with my dad and mum (she would usually be knitting at the same time) and every now and again, my dad would make a remark about a particular part in the film we would happen to be watching at the time. This would vary from things like, "You can tell he's wearing a wig" (he was very paranoid about his hair, ha-ha) to "she's had some work done," or "you can tell they're in a studio" It might seem silly but when you're eight years old, you don't notice things like that and in hindsight, I reckon that's why I am so critical of films now.

At about this time, ITV started showing 'The Six Million Dollar Man' and it's fair to say, I became a

BIPOLAR…..MAYBE?
(Volume Two)

massive fan. Because it was shown relatively early in the evening, my dad would still be in the kitchen talking to my mum and that meant I had the living room all to myself to enjoy the exploits of my bionic hero. To myself that is until 'Top of the Pops' started on BBC1 and then my brother and sisters would come in and turn the channel over. I was the youngest child (still am… funny that) and this always ended up in a big row, with me going into the kitchen to tell my mum what had happened. She would then walk into the living room and tell the others that I was already watching my programme and they shouldn't have turned it over.

"Yeh!" I would butt in, "Top of the Pops is on every single week of the year but 'The Six Million Dollar Man' isn't!"

I did have a valid point and eventually got my way as the others trudged out of the living room with the hump.

"He thinks he's Steve Austin," mocked my brother whilst lifting a cushion above his head, "and can pick up rocks like they were made out of paper!" and then threw the cushion at my head just before leaving the room.

"I've missed some of it now!" I yelled after switching channels but soon caught up with the story and sat down happy again, with the lights off and snuggled on the sofa.

A particular episode was split into two parts and it was the first time the viewers were introduced to Jaime Sommers. She was Steve Austin's girlfriend (man I was jealous) and after a skydiving accident, Steve convinces his boss Oscar Goldman, to save Jaime's life by making her bionic. Eventually, Jaime Sommers got her own TV series and it's fair to say that I was head over heels in love with her. She was played by the actress Lindsay Wagner and I remember having a picture of her stuck to the side of the wardrobe next to my bed and would kiss it every night before going to sleep. Jaime Sommers was the first and only fictitious character I ever had a crush on and each week, I couldn't wait to see the next episode. It wasn't that I was particularly bothered about the plot, I just wanted to see Jaime on the screen and my heart would race every time she appeared and I would spend one hour each week, in heaven! It feels really strange writing about that now and I can almost recall the emotions I was experiencing at the time. The only other actresses to have any kind of effect on me like that are the silent movie stars Janet Gaynor and Louise Brooks, but being more than 45 years later, I no longer feel the need to have their pictures on my wardrobe, let alone kiss them every night. There is something about silent film stars that makes them appear mysterious and alluring… I suppose it's the fact you can't hear them speak which adds to the appeal because you don't know what they sound like.

Anyway, and needless to say, I got even more stick from my brother for watching 'The Bionic Woman' than I did 'The Six Million Dollar Man' and this culminated in him defacing my picture of Lindsay Wagner, by drawing a moustache on her and blacking her teeth out. Yes dear readers, he ruined the thing I cherished the most and I'm not too proud to admit I cried and even now as I write these words, tears are beginning to well up in my eyes (only kidding… or am

BIPOLAR.....MAYBE?
(Volume Two)

I? Yes, I am and it's a shame really)

Purely for the sake of nostalgia (honest guv) I bought the box set of the 'Bionic Woman' when my daughter Nin was about eight or nine and we used to sit down and watch one episode each night before she went to bed.

Nin isn't her real name obviously, it's our nickname for her (long story) and she's really called Leonie. I suggested the name to Debbie while she was still pregnant with her and she really liked it. What I didn't tell her was that the name was a take on Leone (as in Sergio, one of my favourite directors) because I don't think she would have been too happy about naming our daughter after a big fat Italian man.

Anyway, me and Nin used to watch an episode every evening and it was really interesting to see how she responded to it. Jaime Sommers became a heroine to Leonie, much like Steve Austin was a hero to me when I was her age, and I never did tell her that I used to be in love with 'The Bionic Woman'

Because there were only three channels and one TV per household back then, families would all sit down together and watch the same programmes. I have fond memories of all seven of us (mum, dad and five kids) all watching great shows like 'Porridge' and 'Fawlty Towers' and even at that young age, I could tell they were very special. Unfortunately, the whole family watching television didn't last for too long because my sisters Pauline and Ellie were quite a bit older than me, Davey and Jane and by this time, they would go out and do their own thing. My dad could be pretty miserable at times (gawd knows why) so it was brilliant to see him

PART TWO: RELAXATION

literally falling off his seat with laughter when watching Basil Fawlty getting up to his usual exploits. Only a couple of years later, 'Only Fools and Horses' started to be shown on TV and the first few series were really funny and almost in the same league as 'Porridge'... but not quite. The episodes started to deteriorate shortly after grandad died and he was replaced by Uncle Albert. Although good, to me he was obviously acting, whereas with grandad (Lennard Pearce) he seemed so natural and didn't appear to be acting at all. Things declined even further when the girlfriends and wives came into the show (that wasn't what it was originally about) and although John Sullivan was a great writer, the last few series in my mind, were really poor. I think the show suffered because it went on for far too long, unlike Porridge's three series and a couple of Christmas specials, and the fact that 'Porridge' was set in a prison, meant that fashions didn't date the programme at all. Add to that the fact Ronnie Barker was really well spoken in real life (just listen to him read the fake news on 'The Two Ronnies') and then listen to him speak in 'Porridge' and you realise just what a brilliant actor he was. Not once in all of the episodes does he slip up on his London accent and compare that to some of the actors on 'Eastenders' who pronounce their T's when they never actually would in reality... well, there is just no comparison. Ronnie Barker himself admitted 'Porridge' was the best thing he ever made and it didn't hurt that he was accompanied by other fine actors such as Brian Wilde who played Mr. Barrowclough, Richard Beckinsale as Godber, Sam Kelly as 'Bunny' Warren, Tony Osoba as McLaren, Ken Jones as 'Orrible' Ives,

BIPOLAR…..MAYBE?
(Volume Two)

Ronald Lacey as Harris, David Jason (who went on to play 'Del Boy') as Blanco, Peter Vaughan as Grouty and of course the brilliant Fulton Mackay who played… Mr Mackay. With a cast like that and superb writing by Dick Clement and Ian La Frenais, it could never fail to go wrong! It's the same with Fawlty Towers (in my opinion, the funniest sitcom ever made) and the fact they only made twelve episodes seems hard to believe because there is so much going on in each one. As I said before, my dad loved Basil Fawlty but he wasn't a fan of Monty Python at all.

"Load of bleedin' college boys," he would grumble, not accepting the fact that John Cleese was in both shows.

He was also a fan of 'Ripping Yarns' starring Michael Palin, who also wrote it along with Terry Jones, two more members of Monty Python.

I can see why my dad didn't like Monty Python though, the humour was crazy and off the wall, a bit like The Goons who preceded them and to whom my mum is a massive fan.

PART TWO: RELAXATION

CHAPTER 16

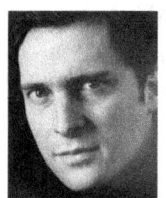

It would be fair to say my dad was strict (especially when compared to this day and age) but my mum could also lay down the law when needed.

It was about half past five on a Thursday afternoon and I still had a few hours to wait until 'The Six Million Dollar Man' came on the telly. My sister Jane had a school friend round for tea and my mum had prepared the table in the kitchen with sandwiches, sausage rolls and Mr Kipling's French Fancies (those colourful little sponge cakes topped with a dollop of buttercream concealed beneath the fondant icing that covered the whole thing) Mmmmm… I could just eat one of them now. There were usually eight in a box and although maths wasn't my strongest subject, I figured that Jane and her mate would have one each, along with Davey and myself and that would leave four going spare. My mum had told us not to come into the kitchen until six o'clock but while she was upstairs, I quickly sneaked in and stuffed two of the cakes into my gob before running back to the living room to digest them. It was now a quarter to six and I could hear my mum coming down the stairs and making her way back into the kitchen. Wiping my mouth and rubbing all the pieces of cake off of my jumper to get rid of the evidence, I sat quietly watching Roobarb (and Custard) while acting all innocent. Just as the news was about to start, I heard my mum calling out my name and assumed it was time for tea. Walking into the kitchen while my brother and sister and her mate were still upstairs, I was then confronted with my mum holding a plate with the remaining six French Fancies on.

"Where are the other two?!" she asked in a stern voice.
"Eh?"
"The other two cakes! There were eight on here a little while ago!"
"But you only get six in a box," I reasoned, hoping she would fall for my deception.
"There are eight in a box and now there are two missing!"
"I dunno where they are," I replied.
"Don't lie to me, I know it was you! There were eight... I know because you were all supposed to have two each!"
Whoops, I hadn't thought of that.
"I don't know mum, I never touched them, honest!" I pleaded in my most convincing voice.
"Yes you did you liar! Davey is upstairs and he hasn't been down!"
"It could have been Jane," I answered, trying to shift the blame onto anyone but myself.
"She wouldn't do that... I know it was you!"
"It wasn't!"
"Was!"
"Wasn't!"
"Yes it was you bleedin' little liar!"! she shouted and

PART TWO: RELAXATION

placing the plate back on the table, she grabbed me by the ear and smacked me on the back of the leg.
It really stung because I was wearing my school shorts but I put on a brave face and yelled, "It wasn't me!"
Smack!
"It wasn't me!"
Smack!
This must have gone on for about ten times, with my leg stinging more and more, and by now and aware of the commotion, by brother and sister and her friend had come downstairs and stood by the kitchen door.
"What's going on!" asked Davey.
"He's eaten two of those fancy cake things and won't admit it!"
"I didn't!"
"Did!"
Smack!
"Alright... I did eat them!" I finally admitted, feeling stupid in front of Jane's friend.
"Right! Now go up to your room... you're not having any tea!"
Davey, Jane and her friend walked past me and sat down at the table and as I stepped through the doorway, I turned back to face my mum and said, "It wasn't me really... I only said that so you'd stop hitting me!"
My mum's face turned red with anger and she yelled, "Come back here you little sod!" but by now I was half-way up the stairs and out of harm's way.
Once in the bedroom I shared with my brother, I shut the door and propped a chair up against the doorknob so my mum couldn't get in (I'd seen it done in a TV show once, where a woman was hiding from the killer)

BIPOLAR.....MAYBE?
(Volume Two)

By this stage, I had lied so much that I was actually starting to believe my own innocence, and being angry with my mum, I decided to run away... and never to return! Rummaging through the bottom of my cupboard, I found my trusty old leather camera case that I'd always treasured (I've no idea why, it didn't even have a camera in it) and decided to use it as a miniature suitcase to pack my most important possessions to take on the long arduous journey with me.

First into the case went my red catapult along with a compass that belonged to my brother, who I figured would be cross if he knew I'd taken it, but it didn't matter because I would never see him again. Next in went some chewy sweets I'd hidden under my bed (they were supposed to be for a midnight feast but never mind) and then a penknife followed by a strange looking shell I'd found on Southend beach. I then removed a pair of laces from some shoes (in case I had to devise some sort of trap to capture an animal for food purposes) and bunged them in, some Swan Vesta matches I'd pinched off my mum, and finally a handful of different sized marbles and one of those see-through rubber balls that were really bouncy (to play with in case I got bored)

I had the whole thing planned out and would use the catapult to kill some prey (such as a pigeon or a squirrel or something) if my shoelace trap didn't work. I would then use the penknife to take the guts out and cut off the head and legs, and finally make a fire to cook the animal with. Who needed mum's home cooking eh? I had the whole situation figured out! Happy with the contents of my case, I secured the lid with the fastener and then placed the strap over my head before creeping downstairs into the living room, while everyone else was still in the kitchen. Carefully sliding open a drawer in my mum's sideboard, I removed the key to the patio doors and quietly opened them before stepping out into the cold dark evening. Slowly closing the doors behind me, I tip-toed round to the side of the house and stealthily unbolted the garden gate before creeping up the drive to the road, and then I was free... freeeee!!!

"I'll show you!" I said to myself and then began to trek down the road until I was at the halfway point.

That's when I spotted my dad's car turn into the road (he'd just finished work) and realised he would see me within the next minute.

"Shit!" I thought, "He'll bleedin' kill me!" and so I turned around and began racing back home, figuring that I could run away any old time.

I just made it to the top of the drive before his headlights could shine on me and by the time he pulled up outside the house, I had managed to shut the garden gate again and run up to the patio doors. Much to my relief, they were still unlocked which meant my mum still didn't know I was missing, and I was then able to lock them behind me, return the key to the drawer and silently climb back up the stairs just as my dad entered the house. Silently closing my bedroom door, I removed my brother's compass from the camera case and returned it to his chest of drawers before tossing the case into the bottom of my cupboard. By now my heart was pounding because I was so out of breath and I could hear my dad's deep voice coming from the kitchen directly below the bedroom. All went quiet for the next couple of seconds but then I heard footsteps coming up the stairs and knew it had to be him. Racing over to the light switch, I turned it off and then ran back to my bed and climbed under the covers just as the door opened. Even though I had my eyes closed pretending to be asleep, I was aware of him standing in the doorway and so I started to snore loudly to add further to my ruse. Expecting him to call my name out at any moment, I couldn't believe my luck when the bedroom door closed and I could hear him going downstairs again. Throwing back the bed sheets, I took off my school uniform and knowing I wasn't going to get any tea, I pulled the covers over myself and tried to go to sleep but it wasn't easy because I was worried what my dad would say the following morning.

Obviously, I must have fallen asleep at some point because it was now morning, and once I'd brushed my teeth and hair (not with the same brush) I got dressed and made my way downstairs to the kitchen.

"Where's dad?" I whispered to Davey as my mum was putting the kettle on.

"He's just left," he mumbled with a mouthful of Shredded Wheat in his gob.

"Did he say anything about last night?"

"No," he said while shaking his head and loading up his spoon again.

"Why didn't he tell me off?! I asked myself and could only assume that my mum had told him that she'd smacked me and he'd figured that was enough punishment.

"You're lucky he didn't say anything," said my mum as she placed a cup of tea in front of me, "but if you ever

PART TWO: RELAXATION

do anything like that again… he won't be so easy on you next time"
I nodded my head slowly before reaching for the Shredded Wheat and muttered quietly, "Sorry mum," and with just those two words, she seemed absolutely fine with me from then on. Well… when I say then on, I don't mean for ever obviously because that would be ridiculous, just until the next time I did something wrong.

BIPOLAR…..MAYBE?
(Volume Two)

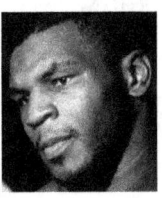

CHAPTER 17

It's funny some of the seemingly unimportant things you remember from childhood, and they reckon having dementia produces similar thoughts. Perhaps thoughts is the wrong word however when describing dementia because calling them thoughts suggests remembering something and as far as I understand it, memories don't actually occur with that condition. Rather they are random triggers in the brain that causes the individual to recognise those so-called thoughts. That then almost makes the human brain even more astonishing than it already is, because it proves that every single memory we have had during our lives is stored somewhere in the brain, like some vast filing cabinet that can be called upon even without the owner's consent. Don't quote me on this, I might be completely wrong… it's just my take on things.
Anyway, during the 1970's there were a series of adverts promoting Unigate milk and the benefits it could have on kid's health. As a visual aid to endorse the milk, red and white striped straws were used as supposed milk thieves that sucked up the milk when you weren't looking. For some reason these adverts were really popular and celebrities such as Spike

PART TWO: RELAXATION

Milligan, Arthur Mullard, Benny Hill and even Muhammad Ali were featured in them but the ads were mostly known for their slogan, "Watch out, watch out—there's a Humphrey about!"

A merchandising campaign went along with these adverts and Humphrey-themed mugs, milk bottles, and straws were available to buy. Try telling kids that today and they would think you'd gone fucking mad but they are the ones who are crazy... I mean, who needs Xbox, PlayStation and Nintendo when you've got a straw to play with? I don't know, kids nowadays.... dunno they're born!

If you were a boy in the 70's, you had to put up with all those crappy teen idols that girls fell madly in love with, such as David Cassidy, David Essex, The Osmonds and The Bay City Rollers (I'm not including The Jackson Five because at least they had some genuine talent) and my sister Jane would carry around her transistor radio with all these bleedin' songs coming out of the tinny sounding little speaker.

I can't stand it when the term boy bands or girl bands is used because a band indicates a group of musicians and most of these people can't even play a note. Also, everything is so much different nowadays and any new groups being formed have such a polished sound about them, almost as if the producers have learned all the mistakes over the years and hired the most talented writers to create the next number one hit. If each new group turns out to be successful with their sterile and mundane songs, the members end up being multimillionaires within a matter of only a few years because the best financial advisers are on hand to

BIPOLAR…..MAYBE?
(Volume Two)

provide their services and we, the adult members of the public, are forced to listen to their songs while they remain prominent in the charts. Don't get me wrong, I wish them all good luck because I'm sure it's not easy getting recognised in the first place but I can't think of anything worse than being recognised wherever you go. The last thing in the world I would want is to be rich and famous… give me the riches anytime but you can stick the fame side of things right up your arse.

My taste in music in the early seventies was far more sophisticated with the smash and surprising hit 'Remember You're a Womble' being among my favourites. My eldest sister Pauline must have hated it, listening to David Cassidy in one ear and The Wombles in the other, especially considering she was into Jimi Hendrix, The Stones and Frank Zappa and the like.

At around about this time, Pauline got a job as a delivery driver working for UniChem, a company that supplied all the pharmacies throughout the country with their orders of medication. As you would rightly assume, no passengers were allowed in the van alongside the driver and to get around this, Pauline would load Davey, Jane, me and all our mates in the back of the van, where we would be out of sight. Letting a load of kids sit amongst boxes and boxes of different drugs was a definite no no, but if Pauline only had to work a few hours in the morning and deliver to say, Southend, then we would all go with her and spend the rest of the day enjoying the sunshine. It was on one of these trips to the seaside where I found the **strange looking shell (you know, the one I packed into my camera case) and I think on that**

PART TWO: RELAXATION

particular day at Southend, it was one of the hottest days of the year. I'm guessing it must have been during the school summer holidays because although it was a week day, the beach was absolutely packed but that added to the adventure somehow.

My mate Richard came with us and I told Pauline that we were just going to the amusement arcade to try our luck on those coin-pusher machines. The place was rammed with people and there was a group of disabled children with a couple of carers, already trying their luck on the machine we wanted to use. The two carers wandered over to another machine and this boy in a wheelchair kindly moved over and said we could have a go. Me and Richard run out of coins in a matter of seconds but the boy in the wheelchair said we could share in his winnings if we helped him put the coins in the slot because it was difficult for him to reach. So, I dropped a two pence coin into the machine and we all watched it fall onto the moving plate and push a whole load of coins forward. Unfortunately, this group of coins balanced over the edge without dropping down and as the kid twisted his wheelchair in frustration, he smashed into the side of the machine and they all suddenly fell off the ledge into our greedy hands. Because the machine was so heavy, it was really difficult for someone to nudge it with their body and try to cheat but the boy's wheelchair gave me an idea and one in which we would all profit. So, we put a few more coins into the slot until another group of them balanced over the edge and then with the kid's consent, I rammed his wheelchair into the machine. Again, all the coins fell but this time and what I hadn't expected to happen, an

BIPOLAR…..MAYBE?
(Volume Two)

alarm started ringing and we all looked over to the big fat man wearing a string vest, sitting in the pay booth. He quickly stood up and looked over in the direction of the alarm but must have spotted the boy in the wheelchair and turned it off before returning to his newspaper.

"Try it again, try it again!" said the boy all excitedly and so Richard dropped some more coins into the slot and away we went again.

I slammed the wheelchair against the side of the machine as hard as I could and this time when the alarm went off, the man left the booth and came wobbling over to us.

"What's going on here?!" he barked, "I hope you lot ain't trying to cheat!"

"I'm sorry," said the boy with an innocent expression on his face, "it's so busy in here I can't move properly and I keep bumping into the machine"

"Then you're gonna have to leave!" said the tubby gentleman and folded his arms across his chest (he would have folded them over his stomach but he was just too fucking fat!)

"You can't do that!" interrupted a woman, who was with her two kids, playing on a pinball machine with a picture of Fonzie from Happy Days on it.

"I can do whatever I like madam, I'm the owner of this establishment"

"It's discrimination, that's what it is!"

"Eh?" replied the man, with the pungent smell of body odour escaping through the holes in his vest.

"You can't tell him to leave just because he's disabled!"

"But I'm the owner…"

PART TWO: RELAXATION

"I don't care if you're the Queen of bloody Sheba, if you make him leave, I'm going straight to the authorities"

This made the man hesitate for a moment and I'm guessing he didn't want the police involved because he had some undercover dodgy dealings going on like overcharging his customers… either that or gun smuggling or something.

"Alright, he can stay," he finally replied and returned to the kiosk.

The woman turned her attention back to her children and the pinball machine, with the voice of the Fonz saying 'Aaaay!" coming from a speaker when her son got a good score.

Checking she wasn't watching us; I rammed the wheelchair into the machine and a whole load of coins came tumbling down the slope. Needless to say, the alarm went off again and giving the boy his share of the winnings, me and Richard quickly scarpered before the man copped on to what was happening and had a chance to throw us out. Before returning to Pauline and the others who were sunning themselves on the beach, we bought ourselves an ice-cream each with our ill-gotten gains and stuffed them as quickly as we could, in the hope my sister would buy us another one when we got back.

I suppose the habit of cheating at games started at an early age with me, and I put the blame solely down to Pauline who was a pro. Whenever we would all play a board game, she'd win every single time and I always wondered how she did it until I caught her hiding some money once, when we were playing Monopoly.

BIPOLAR…..MAYBE?
(Volume Two)

"I'll beat her at her own game," I said to myself and wrote a letter to Waddingtons (the UK manufacturer of Monopoly) asking for a spare set of banknotes.

I can't remember exactly why I told them I needed them (I probably said they got burnt in a fire or dropped down the toilet or something) and much to my surprise about a week late, they arrived in the post addressed to me, and they didn't even ask for any payment or whatever. Needless to say, I was on a winning streak for about the next five games we played until my brother found my hidden stash and the game was (literally) up.

PART TWO: RELAXATION

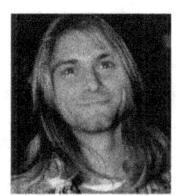

CHAPTER 18

It's fair to say I was a horrible kid and just the sort I can't stand today, 'cos I've become a miserable old git. It seems strange to me now but at the end of our road was Theydon Bois Baptist Church and once a week, me, Davey and Jane would attend Sunday school in the hall next door, even though we don't come from a religious family. I reckon my mum and dad just wanted us out of the way for a couple of hours, so they could have some peace and quiet to themselves and looking back on it now, I can't blame them one bit.

The local Cub's hut was just around the corner from our house and I started going there at the age of eight, much to my displeasure (it sounds like I was a miserable young git too) and was expected to attend just like my brother who was now a member of the Scouts. I hated the outfit we had to wear and to me, it was just another uniform and like being at school again. I couldn't stand going to school as it was, let alone having to go somewhere else as well, especially as it should have been my time off.

I lasted exactly two weeks before being thrown out for bad behaviour and that was absolutely fine by me, but even though I was glad, I still felt it was necessary to

BIPOLAR…..MAYBE?
(Volume Two)

exact some sort of revenge upon the organisation. During the school summer holidays (it always seemed to be the summer holidays and they lasted for ever) me and a group of like-minded kids decided to break into the Cub's hut and steal something, although we had no idea what that would be at the time. The hut was made of wood and was basically a very large shed with windows, but these all had shutters on them when the place was closed and we couldn't figure a way of getting in.

"Let's see if there's a way in up on the roof," I suggested and luckily for us, there was a tree close enough to climb up and cross over to the hut.

Just like its smaller counterpart, the roof was covered with lengths of felt and on the edge of one of the strips, we could see it had raised up slightly which allowed us to pull it back further and expose the wooden slats underneath. Luck was on our side because these slats appeared to be held in place with nothing more than small nails and so removing my penknife from my shorts pocket and opening the blade, I pushed it between two of the slats and began to prise them upwards. Working the blade backwards and forwards entailed a bit of effort and we all took it in turns until finally Richard was able to pull two slats up, and remove the rest of the nails in the process.

I was the first to climb through the gap, which was just wide enough to squeeze through, and dropped down onto a wooden bench that was used by the Akela to show his Cubs simple survival techniques which didn't need to be performed outside. I was then followed by Richard and Trevor, whilst Spencer remained on the roof and started removing another slat so it would be easier for us to climb out. Being as all the windows were shuttered up, it was really dark inside the hut and so Richard took a lighter out of his pocket (which he'd nicked off his mum) and lit it so I could find the light switch. The whole place was suddenly filled with a bright white light when I flicked the switch on and I always remember thinking how quiet and empty the place looked without all the Cubs inside.

"There's nothing to nick," said Trevor as we scanned the interior of the hut.

Realising he was right and anything valuable that could be pinched had obviously been taken home by the Akela, I looked around the large room in the hope of finding something. Suddenly my eyes caught hold of two fire extinguishers; one at each end of the room, but much to my disappointment, I could see they were the only things worth taking.

"But what are we gonna do with them?" asked Trevor once I'd explained my plan.

"I dunno… nick 'em," I replied and started walking over to the first one.

"Why don't we set one off?" said Richard and with that suggestion, we all began to grin widely.

"Just one!" called Spencer from the gap in the roof, trying to be as quiet as he could, "We can take the other one"

"Where to?" I asked while lifting the first extinguisher off the wall and carrying it to the middle of the room, "They're pretty heavy"

"The forest," suggested Trevor, "and we can let that one off there"

With us all agreeing on the idea, Richard and Trevor climbed back onto the bench and I struggled to lift the extinguisher up to them. They both then took a hold of it and began passing it up to Spencer.

"Don't drop it," whispered Richard, "it weighs a fucking ton"

Leaning his top half through the gap, Spencer stretched his arms out and just managed to grab hold of the extinguisher before pulling it towards him and finally out of the gap.

"Be careful Spence," said Trevor, "those things are pressurised"

"Eh? Oh… shit!" replied Spencer and then we heard a rolling sound, followed by two seconds of silence and a muffled thump somewhere outside.

"What happened?" I called out.

"Er… it slipped out of my hands and off the roof"

"Is anyone coming?" asked Richard, looking slightly worried we might not get out of the hut in time and be caught by someone.

"I can't see anyone," whispered Spencer, "but you better come out of there"

"But we haven't let the other one off yet," said Trevor looking disappointed.

Me and Richard looked at each other and although we really wanted to set the second extinguisher off, we realised it was too risky because someone might turn up at any moment.

"There isn't time." I finally said and climbed onto the bench with the other two.

Richard and me then lifted Trevor high enough for his hands to grasp hold of Spencer's, and he then began to

PART TWO: RELAXATION

pull as we pushed under Trevor's shoes. Finally, he was out of the room and on the roof again and I wondered if I were next, how would Richard be able to lift me on his own, and then how would he get out afterwards. Suddenly, I remembered the Akela using a stool to sit on when he was showing us stuff and so jumping back down off the bench and walking round to the other side, I was relieved to find it still there. I then passed the stool up to Richard and wasting no time, he stood on it and was out of the hut before I even had a chance to climb back on the bench. I don't know why but I felt it was important to turn the light off first (probably because it was instilled into me and my brother and sisters not to waste energy, since that in turn cost money)

There was also a part of me that was glad we didn't set the fire extinguisher off inside the hut and after I was finally dragged back up onto the roof, I replaced the wooden slats and covered them with the felt again.

"What you bothering to do that for?" asked Spencer.

"It might rain and the inside of the hut will get soaked," I answered.

"So?"

I just shrugged my shoulders and we all then climbed back down the tree and struggled with the fire extinguisher, carrying it across the cricket field, along a street of houses and finally into the forest beyond the plain.

"But what do we say if someone stops us?" asked Trevor.

"We'll tell 'em we're returning it to its rightful owner," I replied.

"But they'll ask what we're doing with it"

"Then we'll tell 'em to fuck off," said Richard and with that, we all burst out laughing and struggled with that bloody fire extinguisher until we finally reached the forest.

"Now… now what?" asked Spencer when we finally put it down and struggled to get our breath back.

"This," I replied and slowly getting to my feet, I stood the extinguisher upright, withdrew the pin and pulled the trigger whist pointed the hose at my mates, covering them in white sticky foam.

All that hard work and it was over in less than a minute but as least it was fun while it lasted. Needless to say, they held me to the ground afterwards and wiping the foam off their faces and bodies, covered me in it too. Knowing our mum and dads would go mad if they saw the state off us, we then spent the next hour rolling about in the tall grass of the plain to remove as much of the foam off as possible. We then made our way to the village pond and washed our faces, arms and legs and looked almost as good as new (apart from the grass stains but we were usually covered in them anyway)

PART TWO: RELAXATION

CHAPTER 19

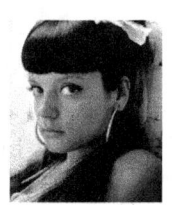

I suppose like a lot of boys (or was it just me?) I seemed to take some kind of morbid fascination in killing insects and during summer, I'd hunt in the garage for an old tennis racquet we had lying about. Armed with my weapon of choice, I would then go into the back garden and wait for a butterfly to flutter by and then took aim.

Swipe! It all happened so fast I don't think it knew what hit him and from being this graceful and beautiful creature, it was now shredded into small fragments like pieces of confetti on a wedding day. I would happily spend a couple of hours swiping away to my heart's content until my brother caught me and went mad. Looking back on it now, I think that's the only time I saw him lose his temper, and he snatched the racquet away from me and stormed inside. He's always been into nature and all that malarky and I was left alone in the garden, surrounded by tiny bits of butterfly wings as if it were me who had just been married.

"I don't need a tennis racquet anyway," I said to myself and waiting until Davey had gone out, went into the kitchen and opened the drawer filled with bits and pieces and odds and sods.

BIPOLAR…..MAYBE?
(Volume Two)

Taking a magnifying glass from the drawer, I went back outside and sat on the patio steps leading down to the garden. Remembering seeing some ants the day before, I was disappointed not to find any, but then I began to bash the side of my fist on the step and sure enough a few seconds later, they started to appear from a crack between two paving stones. Carefully lining the magnifying glass up with the sun, I adjusted it backwards and forwards until the spot of intense light it created was at its most lethal. Then it was just a simple matter of moving the light onto an unsuspecting ant and seeing it frizzle to death and I watched captivated as a small cloud of smoke rose from the corpse (is that the right word for a dead ant?) After killing about twenty or so of the unfortunate Formicidae (the scientific name dear boy… thank gawd for Google) I became bored and decided to try a little variation on the theme. Asking my mum if it was okay to use the phone, I rang my friend Richard's house in Theydon and when he answered, I said I'd be over within the hour.

The walk down to the station took about fifteen minutes and the train journey itself about another half an hour, with a further fifteen-minute walk to Richard's house.

"Fancy killing some ants?" I asked after he opened the door.

"Yeah, but my sister has got the magnifying glass in her bedroom… she's using it to do some homework," replied Richard, thinking we were going to use the most common method of execution.

"We won't be needing that this time, have you got a plastic bag?"

PART TWO: RELAXATION

"I think there might be a few in the cupboard next to the sink"

"If you grab a couple, I've got a plan," I replied and then waited on the doorstep while he went to get to get some.

"I could only take one," said Richard when he got back, "my mum has only got four and she would miss them if I took anymore"

"That should be alright… do you know where we could find some ants then?"

"There's usually some on the step leading into the Cub's hut (yes, that one) and I think there are some red ants too"

So off we went; Richard with the plastic bag stuffed in his pocket in case his mum was watching us from the window, and me with a box of matches I'd taken from the bits and pieces drawer in my mum and dads' kitchen. Just as we'd hoped, when we reached the Cub's hut, there were a load of red ants scurrying about on the wide concrete step and we sat just far enough away so they couldn't sting us.

"What do we need the plastic bag for?" asked Richard as I took the matches from my pocket.

"We can pull the bag apart and then set light to bits of it and watch the melting plastic fall on the ants," I replied and Richard eagerly began tearing the bag to pieces.

Once he had completed his task, I told him to hold a bit of the bag above the red ants and was just about to strike a match, when Richard stopped me.

"What's the matter?" I asked with a confused expression on my face.

BIPOLAR.....MAYBE?
(Volume Two)

"Let's not do it yet," replied Richard, "first let's get some black ants. It's great watching them fight with the red ants"

He then began to slap the palm of his hand on the step about three feet away from the red ants and we waited patiently. Just like back at home, black ants started to appear and carefully picking one up between his thumb and finger, Richard dropped it next to a red ant and we watched spellbound as they began to fight. Whereas the black ant only had its jaws to act as a defence, the red ant was able to use its sting also, and it was fascinating watching the black ant trying to avoid it. Invariably, the red ant finally won the battle but the black ant fought well and could have held his head high in pride at his heroic performance.

"And now for the molten plastic," I said to Richard and seeing as the black ant had lost the fight, we decided to drip some of the melted bag onto a red ant just to be fair.

By now, the black ants had returned to their nest (I think they knew what was coming) and with Richard holding the piece of bag inches away from a group of reds, I struck a match and we watched captivated as drops of liquified plastic fell upon the ants, killing them instantly (at least I'm hoping it was instantly because it must have been really painful)

Another thing I would occasionally do is whack a fly that had made its way into the house with a tea-towel and as long as it was still alive, I'd then stick it in the freezer compartment of the fridge. Like some mad scientist out of a Universal horror film, I would then wait a whole day (hoping my mum wouldn't discover

PART TWO: RELAXATION

it in that time) and then take it out of the freezer and out into the garden. There I would sit patiently as the fly began to defrost in the sunlight, hoping it would reanimate itself and return back to life (they never did, so don't bother trying it yourself)

Then of course there were the times when me and my friends would shoot birds in the garden with air rifles and pistols (this would have been a couple of years later when I was about 12 or 13) and my mate Simon had loads of guns. His mum and dad would let us shoot at targets when they were home but as soon as they went out, the targets were tossed to one side and the killing would commence. I'm ashamed to admit we even used to throw stones at the swans in Theydon Pond but that was probably in an act of revenge after they had chased us across the field, pecking at our legs because we must have got too close to their nests. Anyway, what makes swans so bleedin' superior? They shouldn't have any special privileges above any other creature on Earth, but I still feel guilty all the same.

There was also an occasion where I took aim at the string holding up a bird feeder with an air rifle in Richard's neighbour's garden and I couldn't believe it when it cut on the very first attempt. It put me a little bit in mind of Blondie severing the rope around Tuco's neck at the end of 'The Good, the Bad and the Ugly' although I was only about twenty feet away instead of hundreds.

It's funny how you change when you get older... well, most people do while others start killing larger and larger animals, like cats and dogs, until they end up becoming serial killers and murder people before chopping them up, sticking them in a boiling pot of water and eating them for tea.

I really had to struggle writing about killing those birds because it now almost makes me feel sick, but I realised many years ago that the insects I killed are no less deserving at the opportunity to live a natural life than animals bigger than themselves. Nowadays, if I kill anything by accident, such as treading on a snail, I feel so guilty and terrible that it plays on my mind for quite some time (okay, not days but at least half an hour)

I'm not keen on spiders and if a large one scurries across the floor or along a wall or something, I have to get it out of the house but would never dream of hurting it. So much so that I've bought this special tool to pick spiders up with and it means I don't have to get too close to them. Imagine one of those things people use to pick litter up with but instead of a grabber at one end, it has these soft bristles that form a circular shape and when you pull the trigger, the bristles harmlessly close around the spider and you can then take it outside and let go of the trigger to release it. For anyone who doesn't like spiders, I thoroughly recommend it and you know the spider is unharmed in the process.

Even if I'm weeding in the garden now and I come across a worm, I'll pick it up and throw it safely to one side so as not to harm it, and nine times out of ten, a blackbird close by, who has been watching my every move, will gobble it up, but at least that's part of the food chain and so I don't feel quite as bad. I won't even tread on an ant now if I can help it and find myself constantly looking down when I'm in the back garden. It's almost like I've gone from one extreme to the other,

PART TWO: RELAXATION

and I have to repent for the sins of my childhood but I don't mind cos it makes me feel good when I know I have avoided killing something by mistake. The only things I will now kill are mosquitos, because I just can't stand it when they buzz around my earholes and occasionally the odd fly, but not if it can be avoided. Instead, I'll wait until it's just starting to get dark outside and then turn the light on in the utility room before turning the light off in the kitchen. The fly then usually goes into the utility room and I quickly rush inside and shut the door behind me before turning the light off in that room and opening the side door leading to the garden. Because it is still light enough outside, the fly makes its way through the open doorway before I close the door, happy in the knowledge I didn't have to kill it.

CHAPTER 20

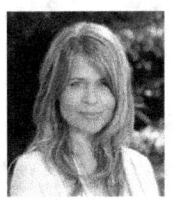

October 1975

Every weekend after Sunday School, my dad would drive me and Davey to the nearby town of Epping and take us to this great model shop called Hancock and Smith. My dad would usually wait in the car or start looking in estate agent windows (he was property mad) while me and my brother would spend ages looking at the hundreds and hundreds of models for sale. Of course, we only had so much to spend (our pocket money and any savings we might have, which in my case was none) so we usually ended up buying either a plane or tank from World War Two at a scale of 1:72. This meant that... let's say, a Spitfire when finished would measure about five and a half inches long and because Davey always had more money than I did, he was also able to buy the correct paints for each of his models (as I'm writing this, I've just looked up the Airfix website and it's brought back so many happy memories)

On this particular occasion I seem to remember my brother buying a Messerschmitt Bf109 with its single prop much like the Spitfire and I bought one of those tanks from World War One, with the tracks visible running around the whole body. As soon as we got home, we would both sit at each end of the kitchen table and commence constructing our models. Whereas I would immediately start pulling each piece of my model off the plastic that held them together, and then squirting way too much glue on them, Davey would carefully remove each piece of his own model and then begin lightly sanding the rough edges with a nail file my mum had given him.

"Mine's gonna be finished well before yours," I said with a grin but my brother simply ignored me and carried on sanding.

About an hour and a half later, my tank was complete and I stared at it proudly, only wishing I'd had the paints to finish it off.

"Aren't the tracks supposed to go round and the machine guns meant to move?" I asked Davey.

"Yep," he replied without looking up, "you've put way too much glue on them"

Shrugging my shoulders, I went into the garden with my tank and began playing with it but I had to hover it slightly off the ground otherwise it wouldn't budge. When it was time to go to bed that evening, Davey had only finished about half of his plane and he told me it would be ready for painting the following night, after we'd gotten home from school. Needless to say, once he had completed the Messerschmitt and spent the next several nights painting it meticulously, the model looked absolutely amazing and even the propeller went found and the wheels moved!

"You see," said Davey, "it's mine that's finished before yours, not the other way round"

BIPOLAR…..MAYBE?
(Volume Two)

"But I finished mine on Sunday," I replied and held it up as if to prove my point.

"You call that finished? Half the bits are missing, the moving parts don't move and it's not even painted"

"So? It still looks like the picture on the box… nearly"

Davey then gently placed his plane on top of his chest of drawers and got into bed.

"And don't go touching it," he said, "now turn the light off"

When Saturday came around and Davey was out with some friends, I thought it wouldn't hurt if I played with the Messerschmitt as long as I was careful. So, I placed it on the carpet next to the bedroom door and then hovered my tank into position and pretended to blow it up. Carefully turning the plane over so it lay on the floor upside down, I started hovering my tank away when the bedroom door suddenly opened.

"Where's Davey?" asked my sister Jane and stared at me with my mouth wide open in shock.

"The… the…"

"What's up with you?"

"The Messerschmitt!"

"The what?"

"The Messerschmitt!" I repeated and pointed down at the ground.

Because the plane had been upside down and at a tilt, one of the wings went under the gap in the door when Jane opened it and now it lay in ruins.

"What are we going to do? He's gonna go mad!" I said, all flustered.

"What do you mean we?" replied Jane.

"Well, you're the one who broke it"

PART TWO: RELAXATION

"Only because you were playing with it by the door. I thought Davey told you not to touch it"

"He's gonna kill me," I mumbled and picking up the pieces of the plane, I placed it back on top of his chest of drawers in a broken heap.

"Do you think he'll notice?" asked Jane.

I nodded my head in silence and stared at what looked like a piece of modern fucking art.

At that moment, mum came upstairs and came into the room.

"What's going on?" she asked.

"John's broken Davey's model plane," explained Jane.

"You're the one who broke it!"

"Is that the plane Davey told you not to touch?" said mum, looking over towards the mess on the chest of drawers.

"Yeh," I replied, "but Jane broke it"

"Let's just say you were both responsible"

"I wasn't responsible at all!" complained my sister, "He shouldn't have been playing with it. How was I to know the stupid thing was by the door?"

After much arguing, my mum said she would take the blame and say she knocked it off the chest of drawers while dusting and then trod on it.

"Thanks mum," I replied, "he would have killed me for sure"

"You're not getting off with it that easy, I'll give him the money to buy a new one and you can miss out on two week's pocket money"

"But…"

"That's the end of it"

Davey ended up taking it surprisingly well, probably

BIPOLAR…..MAYBE?
(Volume Two)

because he couldn't tell my mum off and the next day, my dad took him to Hancock and Smith without me and all I could do was watch in silence as he began toiling on his new model. He actually managed to repair the Messerschmitt (okay it wasn't perfect, but a lot better than one of my efforts) and asked why I didn't go to the model shop with him.

"Mum stopped my pocket money for answering her back," I lied and with that, he got to work with the bloody nail file again.

By far my favourite pastime when playing on my own was with my Corgi toy cars, not the really small ones but the cars that measured about six inches long. I actually didn't have that many but I was definitely content with what I had and would spend hours in the hallway, driving them up and down patterns in the carpet. Every time someone walked through the hallway to get to another room, they would have to step over me and I'd tell them to be careful of my treasured cars. Amongst my meagre collection were Kojak's unmarked 1973 Buick Century Police detective car in dark brown, Starsky's red Ford Gran Torino with the distinctive white stripe (so much for being inconspicuous) a light blue Buick Regal police car with the word 'police' in white letters on the front doors and an orange Mercedes which was very similar to the one Ryan O'Neal destroys in the 1978 film 'The Driver'

I'm sorry if this is all a bit boring for you to read about, but somehow it seems important for me to write down, because the image of me playing with those cars is so vivid in my mind. I would usually play with just two

PART TWO: RELAXATION

cars at a time and place them side by side on a stretch of 'road' on the carpet. Although I wasn't pushing them forwards at all, to me they were travelling at about eighty miles per hour and I would occasionally swerve each car into the side of the other. A picture of the car chase in Bullitt would come to mind, where Steve McQueen's 1968 V8 Ford Mustang GT Fastback was trying to knock the baddies' 1968 440 Magnum V8-powered Dodge Charger off the road (that was a bit of a mouthful) I would sway the cars from side to side as if they were struggling to keep them under control and this simple activity kept me happy for most of the day. I also had the Aston Martin from 'Goldfinger' with all the gadgets that went with it, but I usually didn't include the DB5 when playing with the other cars because I preferred 'normal' vehicles and their real-life settings compared to the escapism of James Bond. Even at an early age, I loved films with good car chases in them but they had to be 'real' and nothing like those ridiculous 'Fast and Furious' films of later years with their CGI laden dependence.

On a different occasion, my sister Jane had gone out with some friends and I went into the bedroom she shared with Ellie (my middle sister)
Jane had this life size doll of a baby which I'm guessing was supposed to be about a year old (so it was pretty big) and its lifelike eyes always fascinated me. You know the sort; when you laid it down the eyes closed and once it was upright again, the eyes opened. I'd taken a Stanley knife from my dad's toolbox and proceeded to cut into the soft plastic surrounding one of

BIPOLAR…..MAYBE?
(Volume Two)

the eyes, as if I were a skilled surgeon. I thought it would be relatively easy removing the realistic orb but I had to hack away with the knife for a good ten minutes before I could finally pull it out of the head and stick it in my pocket. I then tossed the doll to one side, returned the Stanley knife to the toolbox and went back upstairs to my bedroom. Luckily Davey was out (we shared the same room) and taking the eyeball out of my pocket, I held it against my own closed eye and pretended to take it out and examine it. To me, I was Steve Austin in 'The Six Million Dollar Man' and could remove my bionic eye at any time I wished. It was even the same colour as my own eyeball (a kind of gun metal grey) and upon pushing back against my closed 'real' eye, I would pretend I could see for miles, just like my bionic hero. It was only after about twenty minutes or so of playing Steve Austin, that I realised the true extent of damage I had done to Jane's doll and I began to panic.

"What am I going to do?" I asked myself, "She's not gonna be happy"

So, a couple of hours later, my sister got home and when she went upstairs to her room, there was this terrible scream as if someone had been murdered.

"What the bleedin' hell was that?" yelled my dad from downstairs.

"Look… look what he's done!" screamed Jane.

"Who?"

"That bloody John!"

How did she know it was me? It could have been Davey or Ellie or Pauline. Okay, neither of them would have done such a thing and it goes without saying that I was severely reprimanded for mutilating the mannequin

PART TWO: RELAXATION

lying on Jane's bedroom floor. I even had to give the eyeball back so I couldn't play with it anymore but I don't know why Jane wanted it because mum made an eyepatch for her beloved dolly.

Another time, I got home from school and took the transistor radio Jane didn't want any more (well, she wasn't using it anyway) and unscrewing the back, removed the circuit board which was about three inches wide by four inches long. I then stuck it to a piece of card I cut from a cereal packet and placed it around my wrist so the circuit board showed in the gap above the cuff of my shirt.

"Who needs to spend money on 'The Six Million Dollar Man' toys," I told myself and spent the next couple of hours taking cups and saucers out of the kitchen wall units, in such a way that my bionic arm would be visible.

"What are you up to?" asked mum when she walked into the kitchen.

"Just tidying up Oscar," I replied.

"Well don't... now put it all back"

"Affirmative Oscar"

"Who the bleedin' hell is Oscar?"

"Oscar Goldman... he's my boss and gives me missions to go on"

"Yeah well, your mission now is to put all that stuff back," answered mum, "and make sure you do it properly or you'll feel the back of Oscar what's his name's hand!"

"Mum... mum!" called out Jane as she walked into the kitchen.

I was so busy putting all the cups and saucers away

BIPOLAR…..MAYBE?
(Volume Two)

while making the bionic noises of my arm, I failed to hear what she said.
"Have you seen my radio?"
"What radio?" answered Oscar (I mean mum)
"My transistor radio with the black strap"
"No, I haven't… what about you John?"
"My name is Steve," I responded.
"No, it's not, it's John"
"It's Steve and I still haven't seen it"
By this time, Davey had walked into the kitchen and overheard the conversation.
"What's that on your arm then?" he asked and grabbed me by the wrist to show mum and Jane.
"What is it?" said my sister and came closer for a better view.
"It looks like part of your radio," answered Davey and with that, Jane tore my sleeve open to expose the circuit board.
"I hate you, you little brat!" screamed Jane and tore it off my arm before throwing it to the floor.
She then ran upstairs crying while Davey called me an idiot.
"What am I going to do with you?" said mum, "When are you gonna learn to behave yourself?"
Not really listening to what she was saying, I picked up the circuit board / wrist contraption and started to leave the kitchen.
"Where do you think you're going?"
"I'm going to see if Rudy Wells can repair my arm"
"Who the hell is Rudy Wells when he's at home?"
"He's the doctor who helped design my bionics. He really is a genius"

PART TWO: RELAXATION

"GET OUT!"
"Yes Oscar"
"Wait a minute!"
"What is it?"
"Give that to me," said mum pointing to the circuit board in my hand.
"But I've got to give it to Rudy…"
"You're not giving it to anyone and if you think I'm going to let you keep it, you've got another thing coming"
She then snatched the bionic bits and bobs out of my hand, walked over to the pedal bin and dropped them inside.
"Now get up to your room!" she said, "And don't come down unless I call you!"
So, I sloped off upstairs while holding my arm as if the missing electrical and mechanical components were hindering its ability to function correctly.
Later that night when everyone was tucked up in bed, I sneaked downstairs into the kitchen and retrieved the circuit board from the bin, knowing I could only play with it now in secret.
I missed out on pocket money for the next two months for wrecking Jane's radio and promised myself I would behave properly in the future… yeh, right.

A couple of weeks later, I was off school feeling ill (for real this time!) with a cold or something and my mum told me to stay in bed reading my comics while she went to the shops. One of these comics was the now legendary 'Action' which was extremely controversial owing to its violent content and contained such stories as 'Hook Jaw' (a Jaws cash-in but much more violent), Death Game 1999 (a Rollerball cash-in, only a lot more violent) and Dredger, who was a kind of mash-up between James Bond and Dirty Harry (only much more violent)

Needless to say, out of all the 'serious' comics for sale at the time, this was by far my favourite but the original format wasn't to last long before Mary Whitehouse and her cronies ran a campaign to get it banned. They half succeeded and after the first 36 issues were distributed, the comic's storylines became toned down and I soon lost interest. Although issue 37 had already been completed, it was subsequently pulped and replaced by the new 'softer' version.

Anyway, when my mum eventually returned from the shops (this was before she learned to drive) I went downstairs into the kitchen and she gave me a packet of sweets. They were these round chewy spearmint flavoured things, about the size of a one pence piece (the closest I can find to them nowadays are Mentos, look them up) and eagerly opening the packet, I shoved one in my gob. As I said, they were chewy but had a hard coating and before I had a chance to sink my teeth into it, the sweet slipped down my throat and got lodged there. It was really scary because I couldn't breathe, which in turn meant I wasn't able to cough in the hope of dislodging it. Thankfully at that moment, my mum turned around to start unpacking her shopping bags and could see I was red in the face and clearly in trouble. Realising what had happened, she started whacking me on my back with the palm of her hand but the sweet wouldn't move. She must have been really worried (I know I was) and picked me up before turning me upside down, and holding my legs under one of her arms, carried on slapping my back. Still, it wouldn't budge and as a last resort, she sat me on the table and stuck two fingers down my throat. By now I really thought I was going to die, but she somehow managed to remove the sweet and I can always remember seeing blood on her fingers as she took the mint out of my mouth. It's strange how things like that remain in your memories and even to this day, I have never had a sweet like that again.

My job now entails working with adults with learning difficulties and on the occasions when we eat together, some of the guys get something stuck in their throats. It's such a scary thing but luckily, I have managed to clear their throats in one way or another and to say that is a relief, is a major understatement. One of the guys called Michael had something stuck in his throat (although not where I work) but his carer was unable to clear it and he choked to death. It must be such a horrible way to die because there is nothing you can do to try and breathe, and I feel so sorry for his carer who will have to live with that for the rest of his life.

CHAPTER 21

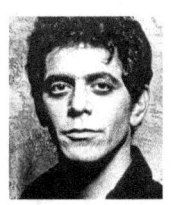

January 1976

I had just turned nine years old and between my birthday on the 11th of December and the Christmas of 1975, we moved from Theydon Bois to Chigwell in what would turn out to be the house I lived in for the next twelve years (on and off)

Me, Davey and Jane were on our Christmas school holidays and Davey had been telling me and Jane about 'Jaws' which he'd just seen, and had been showing at the pictures since Boxing Day. It actually premiered on the June 20, 1975 in America and I think the delay in it being shown in other countries was to attract as much publicity as possible. That tactic certainly worked because 'Jaws' was a huge success all over the world and became what would be known as the first blockbuster movie. A friend of Davey's went to America on holiday with his family in the summer of 75 and we were all jealous because he saw 'Jaws' while he was there and we knew we had to wait another five months.

My mum said that she'd take me and Jane to see it and although scared, I couldn't wait to tell my friends I had watched it before them. It must be hard to appreciate

PART TWO: RELAXATION

nowadays just what an affect 'Jaws' had amongst the cinema going public and ultimately (but I'm sure unintentionally) it ended up causing the mass hunting and killing of Great White sharks to almost an endangered species level. For the period it was released in America to the time it was due to be shown in the UK, we had to make do with teaser trailers at the cinema and even on TV and everywhere you went, there were images of the famous 'Jaws' poster, with the girl swimming and the shark coming up from underneath. This all served to increase our excitement however, so imagine how eager I was as a nine-year-old, to be finally allowed to see it.

The film was given an uncut 'A' certificate by the British Board of Film Classification, which is the equivalent of a 'PG' today and caused quite a bit of controrversy at the time, and in my opinion, still would today. I can always remember queuing in the freezing cold outside the pictures in South Woodford, wearing my dark blue Parka coat with fur lining on the hood and when we finally reached the kiosk, my mum asked for one adult and two children's ticket. The woman behind the counter looked at me and started shaking her head saying, "They shouldn't allow children in to see this film"

I looked up at my mum, who seemed not to have heard her and if it was at all possible, the woman's words added even more to the fear I was feeling. Anyway, we finally took our seats near the back and when the adverts had finished and the lights began to dim, my heart was pounding wildly in my chest. Following the BBFC notice, the Universal logo then came on the screen, accompanied by these faint and strange aquatic sounds. It was then that the music started and without seeing anything but underwater shots and the opening credits, I pulled the hood of my Parka over my head and closed the sides across my face until only my eyes were peering out. That bit was bad enough but when the girl is attacked and pulled under the water, it was safe to say I was absolutely terrified! Throughout the whole film, I must have had that hood pulled over my head for about 70% of the time and for the final half an hour, I don't think I was able to watch any of it at all.

If someone had asked me after it had finished if I'd enjoyed the film, it would have been the wrong question. I knew it had to be good because I was scared witless, which is exactly what the film set out to do, but to say I enjoyed it… noooo! If ever a soundtrack fitted a film more perfectly, John William's simple but brilliant score is just that and even to this day, over 45 years later, whenever that piece of music is played, everyone immediately knows what movie it is from.

That night when I went to bed, I found it impossible to sleep and so anxious was I that I couldn't even get up and go to the toilet. That would have meant putting my foot outside the bed and as ridiculous as it sounds, the bed was almost like the boat in Jaws and the floor around it was the ocean.

It wasn't until 1978 when my dad bought his first video recorder, that I got to see 'Jaws' again (our neighbour lent us a pirate copy of the film and the picture was absolutely awful) but even then, I still struggled to watch it. Then in 1981, it was shown for the first time on UK televisions (it was the highest-rated television programme of the year) and I made sure to record it. By now, nearly six years had passed since seeing at the cinema and being that little bit older, I was no longer terrified and the more and more I watched it, the more I began to realise just what a superb film it was and still is. It almost became a bit of an obsession with me and I would watch it over and over and over again and even though the shark looked fake in some of the shots, I could appreciate how difficult it must have been to make and it was the best they could do at the time. The fact that during production, the mechanical shark kept breaking down actually worked in the film's favour because it isn't on the screen for very long at all (less is more) and it helped enormously that the three lead actors were all at the top of their game. I could write pages and pages about 'Jaws' but don't worry, you won't hear anymore about it, only to say it's my favourite film ever and I've watched it over 70 times.

There was this shop in Loughton called Wilkies that sold all manner of things, including caps for my toy guns and these things me and my mates called Snap Its (although their proper name was Fun Snaps) which consisted of a small amount of rough sand, mixed with a tiny quantity of silver fulminate high explosive and twisted in a cigarette paper to produce a shape much like a cherry. When stepped on, burned, or thrown onto a hard surface, they produced a loud bang similar to that of my cap guns, but the shop also sold boring stuff too, like furniture polish and light bulbs and the like.
Anyway, I'd bought some fake blood from Wilkies at some point and knowing my friend at school had a toy

BIPOLAR.....MAYBE?
(Volume Two)

Great White shark, I asked him if he would like to swap. Much to my surprise he agreed (I definitely got the better part of the deal) and when I got home from school that afternoon, I wolfed down my tea and raced upstairs. I then emptied a shoebox in my cupboard with all the crap I kept in it, apart from three toy soldiers who would act the parts of Brody, Quint and Hooper, as well as two corks I had (gawd knows why) and some string. I then filled the bath up and rolling a bar of soap over and over in my hand to cloud up the water, I put the toy shark in and then the shoebox which doubled as the Orca (the boat in Jaws) With my three heroes now inside the boat, I held the shark in such a way that only his main dorsal fin was prominent above the ocean, with the rest of it obscured by the soapy water.

"Dun, dun, dun, dun... dun, dun, dun, dun," I hummed in the deepest tone I could muster and circled the shoe box as water began to soak into the cardboard.

Pretending to fire the corks, which doubled for floatation barrels, from a line (I tied the string to the corks at one end and onto the shark's Pectoral fins at the other) the three men watched as the corks slowly disappeared below the surface.

It was perfect because the box was slowly starting to sink just like in the film and finally after Hooper went down in the cage (I put him on the bathroom floor temporarily) the shark came bursting out of the water and gobbled Quint up. Brody then positioned himself on the highest point of the shoebox and finally took aim with his rifle.

"Smile you son of a..."

KAAAAAABBBOOOOOOOOOOOOOOMMM!!!!!!

PART TWO: RELAXATION

Lastly, as the boat sank completely under the bath water, Hooper rose to the surface and the two remaining men made their way back to shore.

"Hurry up in there!" yelled Davey while banging on the bathroom door, "It's my turn to go in there now!"

"Won't be a minute!" I replied while pulling the plug in the bath and watching as the saturated shoebox finally became visible again.

When all the water had eventually drained away, I took hold of the water-soaked box and along with the three soldiers and the shark, grabbed it in both hands and unlocked the door.

"About time," said my brother, "what have you got there?"

"Oh nothing," I replied and as I made my way back to the bedroom to throw the sodden mess in my wardrobe, I could hear Davey moaning about the soap scum and bits of cardboard left behind in the bath.

"Use the shower head to wash it all away," I said and then went in search of another box to use the next time I played 'Jaws'

Another weekend and another visit to Wilkies, but this time with my friends and we each bought a box of twenty Snap Its. We then spent the rest of the day walking up and down a busy Loughton Hight Street, throwing the small white bags onto the ground just behind the person in front of us. It was really funny watching the bag explode with a loud bang right by their feet and seeing them jump in the air with fright. Then, as they turned around to see who was responsible, we would quickly turn and pretend to be looking in a shop window. All my friends used up their

Snap Its within a couple of hours but I saved four because I had a great idea how to use them when I got home. Davey was out and only Jane and my mum were in when I walked into the kitchen, and this couldn't have worked out better for me if I had tried. Pretending to use the downstairs toilet, I lifted up the lid and seat and then carefully placed the four Snap Its on the rim of the toilet bowl, so they lined up with the rubber seat buffer things. I then gently lowered the seat and lid back down again and went into the living room to watch TV. Making sure I had the sound down so I could listen out, I hoped it would be Jane who used the toilet first, but alas, this wasn't meant to be. It was my mum who chose to sit on the karzy that fateful day and the relative silence of a Saturday afternoon was abruptly shattered.

BANG!

"I'll kill him! I will… I'll bloody kill him!" screamed my mum and so I made quick my escape and ran upstairs before she could get her hands on me.

"What was that noise?" I heard Jane calling out from below.

"That little sod almost blew the toilet up… and me with it!"

Thinking about it, I was lucky my mum didn't suffer from a heart condition because what with the confined space and tiled walls, and the echo chamber of the toilet bowl, the resulting explosion must have been absolutely deafening!

"It's those stupid banger things he keeps buying," said Jane, "they're such a waste of money. You'd think he'd buy something useful instead"

To my sister they may have been stupid, but they gave

me immense pleasure and I will always look back fondly at the time I almost destroyed the downstairs lavvy.

"Well, he won't be getting anymore pocket money out of me for the next few weeks, that's for sure!"

And so, my mum was as good as her word and I remained penniless (again) for nearly a month, but just the thought of her sitting on that toilet made it all worthwhile.

Then of course, there was the time I stretched cling-film over the toilet bowl so it was invisible, but the less said about that, the better.

CHAPTER 22

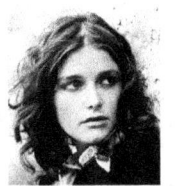

Chigwell 1981

As I mentioned in the previous chapter, 'Jaws' was (and still is) my favourite film and so it goes without saying that the video tape I had of it, was my most prized possession. I'd cut out all the adverts while recording it and wrote not only the title of the film on the tape, but also the duration and certificate (because I'm a sad fucker)

As well as being pretty strict, my dad could also be really miserable (I've no idea why) and when he was in one of his bad moods, he wasn't nice to be around. I remember sitting at the kitchen table doing my homework one Saturday afternoon and he really started having a go at me. By now I was fourteen years old and so my days of misbehaving were behind me, and I was genuinely trying to get on with the homework (shock, horror)

He started calling me spoilt (I'm guessing cos I went to a private school, even though I didn't ask to go to one) and then he swiped all of my school books off the table and onto the floor. Because Epping School was out of our catchment area (the school where my brother and sisters had attended) and the school nearest to the house

PART TWO: RELAXATION

in Chigwell was rubbish, I was sent to Loughton instead.

Years later, when me and my wife were thinking of moving, the idea had occurred to us that we'd relocate to somewhere quite a distance away, because property prices were cheaper. This meant that our kids would have to change schools however and, in the end, we just couldn't take them away from their friends and so decided to move somewhere local. I'm not saying my mum and dad didn't care about me moving away from my mates, it's just that they were always trying to own a bigger and bigger house, to the detriment of anything else.

Anyway, my dad stormed out of the room and I started picking up all my school books before putting them back on the table. Sitting down and trying to forget what he'd done, my dad came back into the kitchen again, but this time with my 'Jaws' tape in his hand. He took it out of the box and began smashing it on the side of the table (I'm guessing to try and break it in half) but when he had no luck doing that, he lifted up the plastic flap, started pulling out lengths of tape and snapping it in two, before throwing it on the floor and marching out of the kitchen.

"What have I done?" I asked my mum when she walked in the room, but all she could do was shrug her shoulders.

Putting my homework away, I took the broken tape up to my bedroom, put on my trainers and quietly left the house so my dad didn't hear me. My eldest sister Pauline lived in a flat in Woodford with her husband Steve and I decided to walk to their place and ask if I could spend the night. When I arrived at the flat, my sister wasn't there but Steve invited me in and made me a cup of tea. Telling Steve what my dad had done (he knew what he was like) I decided not to ask him to stay but instead waited until Pauline got back. When she did finally return, I explained everything but to my surprise, she wouldn't let me spend the night (I'm guessing because she didn't want to be seen as taking sides)

My mum ended up driving to Pauline's and brought me home while explaining in the car that dad had calmed down. Thinking back on it now, I wonder if my dad suffered from bipolar but if he did, I certainly didn't see the 'high' mood swings. I'm literally just thinking about this now but when he was going off on one, maybe that was his way of showing a 'high' episode, because everyone is unique and show their feelings in different ways. If he did have bipolar, I don't think he or any of us knew about it because he never went to see a GP or anything like that, and we all accepted that was just the way he was.

When we got back to the house, my mum went into the kitchen to start cooking dinner, while I went upstairs with some Sellotape and scissors. Cutting off a strip of the sticky tape about an inch long, I then lifted the flap on the video tape and tidied up the two snapped ends with the scissors. All I had to do then was to join the ends together with the Sellotape, wind the spools to tighten it all up and then go downstairs to see if my handiwork was successful. By now we had two video recorders because the first one was starting to play funny and that one was kept in the dining room (which me, Jane and Davey used as a TV room) The newer machine was in the living room and was the one my mum and dad used for themselves. What my dad didn't realise was that the video head drum on the older machine had become dirty owing to the constant use it received. In order to rectify this problem, I removed the cover off the VCR and wiped the head with an alcohol based cleaner and once I'd put everything back, it was as good as new!

So, I went downstairs and much to my relief, my dad was in the living room with the door pulled shut. Creeping into the dining room, I then put the tape in the machine, turned the TV on, rewound it for a couple of seconds and crossed my fingers. Trust my dad to have snapped the tape just when Brody, Quint and Hooper set out on the Orca, and where he'd scrunched it up, the picture went all funny but my repair job seemed to have done the trick and a short while later, the picture became clear again.

When we were all kids, we were lucky enough to go on holidays to Portugal and stay in a great big villa my uncle owned. I say we were lucky but when my dad was in one of his moods (which was quite often) the whole experience wasn't pleasurable in the slightest and all we wanted to do was go home. Anyway, by this stage my brother and sisters had grown up enough that they didn't have to come anymore and that meant it was just me, along with my mum and dad. We went out for a meal one evening and sure enough, dad had the right hump again. During the whole meal, he kept calling me spoilt (it seemed to be a recurring theme) and when it was time to pay the bill, he stood up and told my mum

BIPOLAR…..MAYBE?
(Volume Two)

to go with him and said, "Let him pay for the fucking meal"

I was only fourteen for fuck's sake and didn't have a penny (or escudo) on me and all I could do was sit there alone at the table, with all the other customers looking at me. About a minute later, my mum returned with some money for me to pay the bill and told me she would be outside. I was cross with her because she didn't stand up for me but looking back, I'm guessing she didn't want to cause a scene and make matters worse. It's fair to say I didn't enjoy that holiday in the slightest and couldn't wait to get back to England and see my friends.

I still don't really know why my dad was always picking on me and calling me spoilt, but I guessed his own childhood had something to do with it. He would constantly tell us how poor his family were when he was a boy and I can understand that, but why take it out on me when I had done absolutely nothing wrong? Maybe it was to get his own back for the things I did when I was younger… who knows?

Then there was the time me, Jane, Davey and my mum were eating our dinner at the kitchen table with my dad and he was really in one of his rotten moods. I make it sound like he was always like that but he wasn't; only 99.9% of the time (okay, that's an exaggeration) and on this occasion, he was having a go at mum for one reason of another. Jane had just gotten home from work, as had Davey and my dad, but I was still at school at the time. My dad would often call Jane 'a little Spitfire' because she wouldn't take any nonsense and would stand her

PART TWO: RELAXATION

ground, and this time was no exception. She put her knife and fork down and defending mum, called dad an ignorant pig and a bully. I had to cringe at those words and would never have had the guts to say them myself, and I looked at dad to see him going red with rage. The kitchen was in kind of an L shape and when Jane stood up and walked around the corner out of sight, dad threw his knife and fork down and pushed his chair back. He then stormed into the part of the kitchen where Jane was, and me, Davey and my mum could hear him starting to smack her.

"Get off! Leave me alone!" yelled Jane out of sight, and I looked at my brother (who is five years older than me) and couldn't believe he was just sitting there.

It was only later I realised Davey was scared of our dad (as we all were) but even then, I still think he should have done something.

I was left with no choice but to intervene myself and so I stood up, went to where Jane and my dad were and grabbed him from behind so he couldn't move his arms. Obviously, he was much stronger than me and so I had to be quick and yelled out, "Run Jane!" and watched as she bolted out of the kitchen and upstairs to her bedroom.

I then let go of my dad and pushed him forward, before racing up to the bathroom and locking myself inside. Seconds later, he started pounding on the door and telling me to open up but I refused and he finally went back downstairs to finish his dinner. I waited a good hour before going downstairs again and thankfully by that time, he'd calmed down and went into the living room. It feels kind of wrong writing all these things

BIPOLAR…..MAYBE?
(Volume Two)

about my dad because he died in the December of 2009, but in order to describe my childhood, I don't see that I have any other choice. Okay, I suppose I could not write anything at all but then there would be no book (that would save on paper I hear you say) and it's safe to say, out of me, Davey and Jane, I took the brunt of most of my dad's bad moods.

Ahhh… happy families!

CHAPTER 23

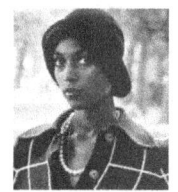

1986

Me, Rob, Ed and Jerrod went to this nightclub in Tottenham called The Ritzy on a Saturday night and because Ed's dad had just bought a new BMW 3 series and he was allowed to drive it, we didn't need to get a cab. If you asked me, Ed was mad 'cos I'd much rather have a drink than drive a car but that was his choice and we certainly weren't complaining. The building itself was massive and although it was a crap name, the club was actually really good and they played some great music. The only real problem with it was the area because it was pretty rough and we found that out for sure when it was time to go home later that night. Although parked up in a proper 'official' car park, someone had smashed one of the back windows to the BM and had tried to take the stereo without success. Understandably, Ed was pretty pissed off about it, so it came as a real surprise when the next week, not only had the window been replaced, but Ed drove us to the same place again. The building was constructed in 1910 and initially served as roller skating rink before being converted to an ice rink. After World War One, its popularity as an ice rink declined and so it was

BIPOLAR…..MAYBE?
(Volume Two)

converted into a dance hall called the 'Tottenham Palais' and it stayed like that for many years. It wasn't until the 1980's that it became known as the Ritzy Nightclub, but its days were finally numbered and it was demolished in 2004 after serving as a bingo hall.

So, we went back there the following week and I must have pulled the ugliest girl in the whole building (sorry if you're reading this) and we were the last ones on the dancefloor at the end of the night. Oh gawd, I feel sorry about saying that now and I'm sure you have grown into a beautiful woman, but you've got to admit you were dodgy looking back then. Anyway, I must have come to my senses because I left with the others and when we got to the car, the exact same window had been smashed again.

Ed's dad had a temper on him and I didn't envy Ed having to explain it to him again, and on the way home, we stopped at a burger stand on the side of the road. It was a converted trailer and me and Ed were the first to get served and while we ate our burgers and watched Robert and Jerrod waiting at the counter, I noticed that the large wooden hatch above their heads was held in place with nothing more than a golf club. Thinking that Ed needed cheering up because of the smashed window incident, I knocked the golf club out of the way and the hatch came swinging down and bashed into the back of their heads. As the lights in the trailer flicked off and on over and over again, Rob and Jerrod's heads were forced forwards and they smashed their faces into the metal counter in front of them.

"What the fuck do you think you're doing?" yelled the man as Ed burst out laughing, and I was happy in the fact I had lightened his mood.

"I'm sorry mate," I said apologetically, "my arm slipped and I knocked the golf club by accident.

"Don't give me that load of old bollocks!" he replied, "Go on… fuck off the lot of you!"

The man had just put Rob and Jerrod's burgers on the counter before the hatch came down (which was handy because it softened the blow to their faces hitting the counter) and grabbing their grub, they ran to the car with tomato relish all over their boats. Me and Ed were already in the car at this stage and with the burgers in their hands, Jerrod and Rob jumped in the back without paying and the 3 series wheel spinned away. While this was happening, the man had gotten out of the trailer and threw the golf club at us. It hit the car where the window had once been but luckily it didn't find its way inside, and we all watched the man jumping up and down in anger as the car disappeared into the night.

"I don't think we'll be eating there again anytime soon," said Ed and turned on the stereo full blast.

Late July, 1987

I'd been seeing my future wife Debbie for the last ten months and we decided to go on holiday to Portugal for three weeks. For the previous three years I had gone away with my mates (to Fuengirola in Spain, San Antonio in Ibiza and Playa de las Americas in Tenerife) and I hadn't been to Portugal in four years. The town of Albufeira had always been a busy place to visit but I suggested to Debbie that we stay in the hotel Sol E Mar because it was in the old town (so nothing would have changed) and I was familiar with it. The idea was that

BIPOLAR…..MAYBE?
(Volume Two)

we could have the best of both worlds, with the new area of the town (which had now grown into a city) being somewhere we could travel to at night and the old part being where we stayed. The Sol E Mar was the hotel where me and my mum and dad went for that meal and my dad stormed off, telling my mum I should pay for it, but even so, I still had happy memories of the place and thought it would be strange staying there, seeing as we had spent so much time at the hotel in the past.

Although I'd had a really good time with my mates on those three other occasions, this turned out to be the best holiday I ever had and Debbie agreed too (Gawd knows what she'd say about it now!)

The Sol E Mar has a really unusual design wherein there is only one side to the building, except for the top floor, which on most hotels would be the bottom floor (confused yet?)

So, walking into the entrance to the building, you would think it was only one storey high, but stepping past the reception into the bar area, you were faced with all these patio windows. Upon opening one and stepping out onto a balcony, you realised that you were on the top floor and all the hotel room's balconies faced onto the sea, going down a cliff face that it was built into and directly onto the beach.

My uncle Bo had lent me a spare set of keys to his villa (which was about twelve miles away) and he wasn't due to go out there until a fortnight later, so we had two weeks of being able to use the pool and all the facilities that went with it. This was before me and Debbie had any commitments, such as kids and a mortgage, and therefore, we had loads of spending money and let's face it and like it or not, without money you just can't do very much. We hired a car for the full three weeks and had such a laugh, driving up into the mountains and visiting places I had gone to as a kid.

About ten miles from the villa is the old town of Silves which used to be the capital of Portugal many years before and I remember when we visited there in my childhood, I was bored to tears because it wasn't a touristy town. It was only on this holiday with Debbie that I fell in love with the place and the sight of the Moorish era castle (9-12th century) positioned high up on the hill and dominating the skyline when you turned a bend in the road, really was something to see.

(Sorry if this is starting to sound like a tourist brochure, I'm not getting a commission… honest!)

The villa is near to Alcantarilha Station, which is practically in the middle of nowhere and calling it a station is almost an exaggerated description. It's one building that looks like it could have come straight out of a Sergio Leone 'dollar' film and the trains that used it were these big old diesel engine things with carriages that really did look like they'd come out of a western. There is a lovely port city called Portimão, with its fishing boats and sea-food stalls, and we could have easily driven the forty-minute journey there, but chose to take the train instead, so we could take in the scenery on the way there (you really need to take the train journey yourself to appreciate what I'm going on about) On the third week of our holiday, my uncle Bo and aunt Annie arrived at the villa and me and Debbie decided to pay them a surprise visit. Whenever Bo would return

BIPOLAR…..MAYBE?
(Volume Two)

to work after being in Portugal, he looked ridiculously brown but would always say the same thing, "I never lie in it"

So, imagine my surprise when we pulled up outside the villa and I stood on the wall to look down into the pool area. It was at the hottest point in the day and he was stretched out on the sun-lounger, soaking up the rays for all they were worth. When he finally spotted us, we went into the villa and both Bo and Annie were really friendly towards Debbie, although he did say to me that he thought I'd only booked a two-week holiday (Bo was the boss of the family business)

We stayed for about an hour before finally making our way back to the hotel and after being in our room for a short while, the telephone rang and the lady said Bo was on the line. He rang to invite us out for a meal in a lovely restaurant I'd been to when I was younger, and it was so nice to spend that time with them both. Me and Debbie ordered Cataplana, which is this delicious seafood dish a bit like stew and is cooked and served in this big metal bowl of the same name. You can only order it for a minimum of two people and if you like your fish, you'll be in heaven. Man, it's lush!

When I got back to England and Bo returned about three weeks later, he gave me a pay rise (I didn't even have to ask for it!) and I'm guessing he felt that I'd matured somewhat, after seeing me and Debbie in Portugal.

It was only a few years later when Annie fell seriously ill and was hospitalised, and a short while after that, Bo sadly passed away. His funeral was quite a small affair and when we all went back to his house afterwards, the phone rang and it was the hospital to say that Annie had died. Even though she had been ill, it was still quite a shock and I'm so glad we spent that time with them in Portugal, even if it was only for a few hours and that's the way I shall always remember them both.

BIPOLAR…..MAYBE?
(Volume Two)

PART THREE: RECREATION

PART THREE: RECREATION

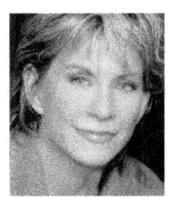

CHAPTER 24

When I was about seven or eight and we still lived in Theydon Bois, Pauline would tell me, Davey and Jane ghost stories on a Friday night just before we went to sleep (and practically guaranteed we each had a nightmare when we finally nodded off)
Pauline would sit on the end of Davey's bed and Jane would get in with me because we were both that bit younger and scared (but in a good way)
I can't remember Pauline reading from a book so I'm guessing she made the stories up and although I've forgotten most of them, there's one particular story that has stayed with me all these years later. Listening to it now, I don't find it scary in the least but you have to remember I was only young and Pauline was always great at doing different voices and stuff. This is the story as far as I can recall it… I hope it doesn't give you nightmares.

Once upon a time there was a little boy called Johnny who lived in the countryside, in a tiny cottage, and was playing with his toy soldiers upstairs in his bedroom. He lived alone with his mother and one Saturday morning, she came up to his room and gave him some money to go to the shops.

Johnny always knew when his mum was walking up the stairs because he would hear them creak under her weight, and he waited for her to open the door.

"Be a good boy Johnny and go to the butchers," she said upon entering the bedroom, "and get me some liver for our tea"

"Okay," replied Johnny and put the bag his mother gave him in his pocket before taking the money she handed to him.

"There's a bit extra there," she explained, "you can get yourself some sweets as well"

"Thanks mum!" said Johnny and racing downstairs, he put on his coat which was hanging by the door and then went outside before jumping on his bike and riding towards town.

In order to take a short cut and save time, Johnny decided to ride through the cemetery even though it scared him, and he peddled as fast as he could while staring at the ground so he didn't have to look at the gravestones. Staring ahead briefly, Johnny could see the open gates at the other end of the cemetery, but just as he was about to peddle even faster, the chain on his bike slipped off the cog on the back wheel and he slowly wheeled to a stop. Climbing off the bike and putting the kick stand in position, Johnny got a handkerchief from his pocket and began to feed the chain back onto the cog.

Hearing voices in the distance, he looked between the spokes of his wheel and could see a group of people slowly walking away from a grave site, before two men armed with shovels approached the large mound of

PART THREE: RECREATION

earth next to it.

"Let's go for our lunch before filling it in," said one of the men and Johnny watched them walk off in the opposite direction.

At that moment, a cold breeze swept through the cemetery and Johnny could feel goosebumps rising on his arms.

"I'm surrounded by all these dead people," he told himself and after successfully reattaching the chain to the cog, he climbed back on his bike and peddled as fast as he could through the open gates.

Once he finally arrived at the shops and was about to walk into the butchers, Johnny couldn't help but notice the sweet shop next door and decided to get himself a bag of Tooty Frooties before buying the liver for his mum. Giving the old lady the money for his sweets, Johnny then went next door to the butchers, but upon asking for the lb of liver his mother asked for, he realised he didn't have enough money left.

"What am I going to do?" he asked himself, "I've spent too much money on the sweets"

Knowing how angry his mother would be if he didn't come back with the liver, Johnny started to panic and stepping out onto the pavement, he began to eat all of the Tooty Frooties, one after the other.

"I can't go home without it!" he told himself and, in an effort, to calm himself down, he walked back into the sweet shop and bought a bag of Lemon Drops.

"I definitely haven't got enough to buy the liver now," Johnny said out loud while climbing back on his bike and then started peddling back home while trying to figure out what he'd tell his mother.

BIPOLAR.....MAYBE?
(Volume Two)

Riding out of town, Johnny was just about to pass the cemetery gates and take the long way home, when an idea came to him.

"That body those two men were about to bury," he thought, "maybe they're not back from their lunchbreak yet?"

Not entirely sure what he planned to do, Johnny began to ride his bike back through the cemetery again, and could see the mound of earth with two shovels sticking into it. Climbing off his bike next to the open grave, Johnny looked around to make sure the coast was clear before grabbing one of the shovels and jumping down on top of the coffin. He barely had enough room to place his feet on the earth next to the wooden box, and using the shovel like a crowbar, pushed the blade between the base and lid and began to prise it open. The nails made a loud squeaking sound as they were pulled out of the wood and when Johnny checked that no one was coming and had enough of a gap, used his hands to pull the lid up and lean it against the side of the hole. Staring down inside the coffin, Johnny looked on in fear at the body of a smartly dressed man, with his hands folded across his chest.

Holding the shaft of the shovel in both hands, he closed both his eyes and brought the blade down with tremendous force, causing it to slice into the man's clothes and body. Acting as quickly as he could, Johnny took the bag out of his pocket, grabbed the man's liver in both hands and pulled it out of the corpse before placing it in the bag and closing the coffin lid again. He then climbed out of the hole and was relieved that nobody had spotted him as he hung the bag over one of

PART THREE: RECREATION

the bike's handles. Johnny then started to ride as fast as he could away from the grave before anyone could spot him.

The cold breeze appeared again and swept through the branches of trees, with the sound of leaves rustling like a distant whisper.

"Johnny... Johnny... Johnny," came the faint sound.

"It's only your imagination," thought Johnny but peddled faster nevertheless, wanting to get out of the cemetery as soon as possible.

Arriving home twenty minutes later, Johnny climbed off his bike, gave his mother the bag with the liver inside and started to make his way upstairs.

"What took you so long?" she called out from below.

"The chain came off my bike," he replied but decided to leave the rest out and was pleased he didn't have to lie to her.

"I'll call you when dinner is ready but it won't be for a couple of hours yet," said Johnny's mother and disappeared into the kitchen.

Deciding to play with his soldiers again, Johnny lay face-down on his bed and pretended they were shooting each other during a battle in the Second World War.

"Johnny... Johnny... Johnny," said a whisper, barely audible over his own breathing.

This whisper caused Johnny to look up at the oak tree outside his window, but there didn't appear to be any movement and the leaves remained motionless.

"It's all in your mind again," he told himself and turned his attention back to the toy soldiers.

"Johnny... Johnny... Johnny," came the whisper again but this time it was followed by a creak and Johnny recognised the sound as coming from the wooden staircase outside his bedroom door.

His heart began to pound inside his chest and he wanted to call out to his mother but was afraid that in doing so, it would alert whoever was on the staircase, of his presence.

"Johnny... Johnny... give me back my liver," said a man's voice, much clearer this time and was followed by the sound of someone climbing up the stairs.

Clump, clump, clump... "Give me back my liver... I'm coming to get you Johnny... I'm coming for my liver"

Clump, clump, clump.

Judging by the noises outside his door, Johnny could tell whoever was out there, must have been about halfway up the stairs and getting closer with each passing second.

"My liver Johnny... give me back my liver"

Clump, clump, clump.

"If you don't give me back my liver Johnny, I shall take yours"

Suddenly the noise on the staircase stopped and Johnny guessed whoever it could be, must now be standing on the landing with its carpeted floor.

"Johnny... Johnny"

The voice was now so clear, Johnny knew it must be close and this was confirmed when he looked down at the gap under the door and saw a shadow appear against the strip of light.

Unable to take his eyes off the shadow, Johnny swallowed hard and was about to ask who was there, when, BANG, BANG, BANG!!!

The pounding on the door was so loud that Johnny

nearly jumped out of his skin.
"My liver... give me back my liver!" demanded the voice, no longer a whisper but a muffled yell.
"I... I... I have... haven't got you liver," stammered Johnny.
BANG, BANG, BANG!!!
"I need my liver... give me back my liver... I want my liver!"
BANG, BANG, BANG!!!
At that very moment, Johnny opened his eyes and finding himself on the bed, realised that he must have fallen asleep and been dreaming the whole thing.
All was quiet for the next few moments, until suddenly,
BANG, BANG, BANG!!!
"Who... who is it?" asked Johnny, terrified as to what was on the other side of the door.
BANG, BANG, BANG!
"Why won't you answer me?" said Johnny's mother, "I've been calling you"
"Phew... it's only you mum, I think I fell asleep"
"Well hurry up and come down for your tea... your liver is on the table!"

It's funny how I can remember that particular story above any others, maybe because the boy's name was Johnny and I was so relieved to find out it had all been a bad dream... or had it?
BANG, BANG, BANG!!!

CHAPTER 25

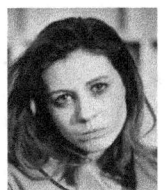

My brother and his mates had a friend called John Smith and if he was a couple of years older than them; I must have been eight, my brother thirteen and John Smith fifteen. You have to imagine that to an eight-year-old, somebody of fifteen was like a man and John created this alter-ego known as Johnny Star, who was this stunt-man extraordinaire and willing to sacrifice his life for the pleasure of his adoring public.

Not so much a stunt but rather a labour of love, Johnny Star assembled a group of minions who would undertake any task he commanded of them, and work began on 'the hole' which as time passed, grew wider and wider and deeper and deeper, until it was eventually about eight foot in depth and resembled a well (but without the little roof and a bucket on a rope)

It was in a small wooded area, close to the Cub's hut and John was like a prison warder, ordering his prisoners to carry on digging and would often call out, "The hole must go on!" to give them some incentive.

I don't actually know what the hole was for but when it was complete (and approved by John) the top was covered over with thin branches and dead leaves, as if it was a trap to capture a wild beast.

PART THREE: RECREATION

"Now what are we going to do?" asked my brother.

"I have an excellent idea!" replied Johnny Star, and ripping one of the sleeves off his jumper, he went and stood about twelve feet away from the hole.

"When I give the word, you tell me to go!" he explained, "And then tell me to jump just as I'm about to fall down the hole"

Everyone looked at each other as if he was crazy but never-the-less, he took his position, tied the sleeve around his head so his eyesight was obscured and then raised a hand in the air.

We all waited in silent anticipation and when he finally lowered his hand, my brother yelled, "Go!" and he began running forward as fast as his legs could carry him.

Nearer and nearer to the covered hole he ran and when he was less than eighteen inches away, Davey shouted for him to jump. Everything seemed to slow down at that point and as Johnny Star leapt into the air, we all held our breath and watched as his feet came crashing down on the branches and leaves. Either my brother had shouted too early or John didn't jump far enough, but he went crashing down into the hole and everything became silent. We all looked at one another for a few moments and then circled the hole and gazed down inside. All that could be seen were loads of broken branches and scattered leaves, with a leg sticking out at one point and an arm at the other.

"Are you alright down there?" called out my brother's friend and after several more seconds of quiet, the branches and leaves suddenly went flying about the place and John stood up.

"Johnny Star is okay!" he called out, "Just a few cuts and bruises. Come back at this time tomorrow and you will witness an even more death-defying spectacle!"

Everyone cheered and someone had to help pull him out of the hole before we covered it over again, in the faint hope that a bear or wolf or something might come along… well, either that or a squirrel and then we all split up and made our ways home.

"What are you gonna do now Johnny Star?" I called out as John walked across the field.

"I have to prepare for tomorrow's stunt kid!" he replied, "But first I'm going home for my tea!"

As me and Davey walked home, I decided to draw a poster celebrating the exploits of Theydon's most daring stuntman and couldn't wait to show it to my hero the next day.

"He's so brave!" I said to my brother, "I could never have done anything like that!!"

"He bleedin' mad!" said Davey, "I wonder what he has got planned for tomorrow?"

After I had finished my tea and had a bath, I went down into the kitchen with some felt-tip pens and a sheet of paper and started work on the poster. The main image consisted of Johnny Star wearing a golden cape blowing in the wind as he jumped over the hole on a fancy looking motorbike. The branches covering the hole were on fire and the fact that never happened and the only bike John owned was of the push variety, didn't seem to matter to me.

JOHNNY STAR… THE BRAVEST MAN IN THE WORLD! read the headline and after colouring it all in with the brightest colours I could find, I went upstairs

PART THREE: RECREATION

to bed but couldn't sleep, eager to show him my artwork the next day.
"What do you think he's going to do?" I asked Davey when he came up to bed about an hour later.
"Who knows," he replied, "he just said to meet him by the Cub's hut at four o'clock"
The following day, I made some finishing touches to the poster, such as adding a few stars to represent his stage-name and when ten to four came, I put a couple of drawing pins in my coat pocket, rolled up the poster and made my way to the Cub's hut with Davey. Johnny Star was already there when we arrived, as well as Davey's other friends, and John had made a black mask which he wore, much like the one Batman wears in the TV series. Unrolling the poster, I showed it to my hero and after laughing out loud, he patted me on the shoulder and said I had done him proud. I then fixed the poster to the side of the Cub's hut with the drawing pins and sat with Davey and his mates on the trunk of a fallen tree.
"And now for my most dangerous stunt to date!" boomed Johnny Star, "I shall need the assistance of a member of the audience"
Nobody offered to help (probably due to the fact they didn't want to risk getting hurt) and so Johnny picked someone at random, which happened to be Davey's friend Steven Anstis. Begrudgingly rising to his feet, he slowly walked over to John and stood next to him, looking terrified.
"Do not be alarmed my friend!" said Johnny, "Your life is not in any danger!"
"What… what do I have to do?" asked Steven quietly.

BIPOLAR.....MAYBE?
(Volume Two)

"If you will observe that tree over there, you can see a car tyre at the base of the trunk"

We all turned our heads in unison and could indeed see a tyre that was sat on top of another fallen tree. From the tyre there appeared to be a length of rope that was tied to a branch, about twenty feet up from the ground.

"Now young man... what is your name?"

"It's Steven, you know it is... I've known you for five years"

"Now Steven, I'd like you to climb up that tree and when you reach the branch that the rope is tied to, begin pulling the tyre up"

"But it might be too heavy," replied Steven, clearly wishing he was somewhere else.

"Too heavy? A fine figure of a man like you! Come, come my good man... do as I ask"

So, Steven began to climb up the tree and as he did, Johnny Star watched from below, with his hands on his hips and waited for him to reach the branch.

"I now want you to start pulling the tyre up and grab a hold of it firmly with both hands!"

Finally, after a lot of huffing and puffing and effing and blinding, Steven was able to hold onto to the tyre and yelled out, "I've got it!"

"Very good young man!" shouted Johnny and then proceeded to lie down on his back, right beside the trunk of the tree.

"Are you ready?!" he finally called out.

"Ready for what?!"

"When I give the word, I want you to let go of the tyre!"

"But... but it will fall right on top of you and you'll beat me up!"

PART THREE: RECREATION

"You have my word that nobody shall beat you up... now do as I say!"
"Do you promise?"
"Yes... I promise!"
I watched in fascination and thought to myself, "Surely he's gone too far this time," but still couldn't wait to see what happened next.
"Are you ready?!" repeated Johnny Star, lying motionless on the ground.
"Yes, I'm ready!"
"Release the tyre!"
"But..."
"Do as I say... release the tyre!"
Steven seemed to freeze for a couple of seconds, which only served to increase the tension and then finally let go of the tyre.
"Geronimo!" he yelled and the rest of us all watched as the tyre fell towards the ground, directly where John was lying.
I almost covered my face but decided against it because I didn't want to miss anything and watched the tyre hurtle straight towards Johnny Star's face. Much to my amazement, he didn't move an inch as the tyre stopped about four inches from his face and sprang back into the air. Down it came again and slowly began to stop still, before John rolled out of the way, got to his feet and took a bow.
"Thank you fans!" he called out. "And thank you to my young assistant!"
After climbing down the tree, Steven took a bow also but just at that moment, someone yelled, "Shit, it's Toby... and he's on the loose!"

BIPOLAR…..MAYBE?
(Volume Two)

Toby was this really vicious mongrel dog which was owned by Mark Bray, who was the youngest son of a notoriously tough family.

We all looked in the direction of the Bray household and could see Toby running across the field and straight towards us, at what looked like a hundred miles an hour. Everyone got to their feet and being terrified of Toby, I climbed up the tree quicker than a rat up a drain pipe and finally stopped when I reached the branch above the one with the rope tied to. Behind me clambered John and I could tell that even with his mask on, he looked petrified.

"If Johnny Star is frightened of Toby… he really must be vicious!" I told myself and then watched relieved as Davey and the rest of his friends climb up the tree next to the Cub's hut.

When John reached the branch with the rope tied to it, he hung on tight and we both watched Steven Anstis finally begin to climb the tree. He just managed to climb high enough and out of reach before Toby arrived and began barking angrily. John then started to swing the rope from side to side and Toby sunk his teeth into the tyre and began swinging as well, with his whole body now off the ground. As John started to pull the tyre up, Toby finally let go and began jumping up and down and snapping at Steven's heels. It must have been really difficult for him to cling on to the tree trunk because there were no branches to hold and when Johnny Star finally grabbed the tyre, he looked down at Steven and said in a menacing voice, "And now you know who your true friends really are"

He then let go of the tyre and it came crashing down on

PART THREE: RECREATION

top of Steven's head, causing him to let go of the tree trunk and fall to the ground below.
"Aaaaaaaarrrrggghhhh!!!" Help me!" he screamed as Toby began to attack him, and all I could do was watch helplessly from above.
Right at that moment and luckily for Steven, Mark Bray came running up and dragged his dog away, before putting a lead on him (I say lead but in reality, it was nothing more than a length of rope)
As Mark began dragging Toby away, Steven climbed to his feet and we all noticed that his trousers were torn to ribbons.
"You're lucky it was only your trousers!" yelled Johnny Star and began laughing.
"Why John, why!" asked Steven with tears in his eyes, "I was your assistant and everything"
"I thought it would be a great end to the act," said John as he climbed down the tree and patted Steven on the back.
"I've got a really good idea Johnny Star!" I shouted, still up the tree.
"Eh... who said that?"
"It's Davey's little brother," said Steven and pointed up towards me.
"I forgot you were even up there. What's your idea then kid?" asked John lighting a cigarette and clearly not interested in what I had to say.
"We could put some food next to the hole covered with branches that we dug yesterday and the next time Toby escapes..."
"We can trap him!" replied John, finishing my sentence for me, "Say... this kid ain't as stupid as he looks!"

"And we could put some spikes at the bottom of the hole…" I continued.
"That's not a good idea," said Davey after he had climbed down the other tree, "Mark might be chasing him and he could fall down there too"
"Oh, I don't know," replied John as he took off his mask, "it'll be like killing two birds with one stone. I mean, what with that fucking dog… they're both like a couple of wild animals and we'll be doing the world a favour, putting them out of their misery!"

PART THREE: RECREATION

CHAPTER 26

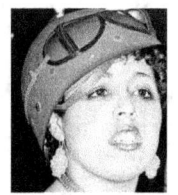

1982
My friend Chris's mum and dad lived in this beautiful little two-bedroom cottage, which was situated on the highest point of Loughton and overlooked Epping Forest, with the thousands of trees sloping away down into the valley below. Chris was an only child and his mum and dad would often leave him alone while they spent weekends on their 45-foot motor boat, but far from feeling lonely, I think he really enjoyed his independence. The area is so picturesque and only a short distance away in the forest is where the Robin Hood section of the film 'Time Bandits' was being made. Chris said he witnessed the filming of this scene and even got to say hello to John Cleese, which was pretty cool (although I'm not really a fan of him nowadays)
Anyway, it was on one Saturday evening and me and my mate Rob were really bored, with nothing to do (this is before we started going into pubs) and knew Chris would be at home with his girlfriend. Both of us didn't like her very much and the feeling was very mutual and so we decided to make an assault on the cottage as an act of retribution. Both of us were dressed in dark

colours and being winter time, we had our coats on and pulled the hoods over our faces to help conceal our identities. Just getting to the house was a real slog because it was all uphill and there were no streetlights, so all we had to guide us was the light of the moon. Chris's bedroom was at the back of the cottage and scaling a metal drainpipe next to the garage door, we tip-toed across the roof (which was flat above the garage, with the rest being thatched) and reaching the rear of the house, Rob said he would climb down first into the back garden.

"Watch this," whispered Rob, "I could have been a Ninja"

Carefully turning round and getting down on his knees, he was just starting to lower himself down the back of the house, when he lost his footing and slammed both his feet against the glass patio doors. All of a sudden, floodlights came on everywhere and the deafening sound of an alarm bell started ringing in the midnight air. Using all my strength, I pulled Robert back up onto the roof and then we raced to the front but misjudged where it stopped and ran right off the end. With us both lying on the ground in a jumbled heap and panting for breath, the front door suddenly opened and in the most threatening voice he could muster, Chris called out, "Who's there?!"

By some miracle, me and Rob hadn't broken any bones and scrambling to our feet, we ran off down the lane and could hear Chris's girlfriend saying in the distance, "I bet it's those two friends of yours... I don't know why you hang around with them, they're a couple of idiots and are so immature!"

PART THREE: RECREATION

Once we were out of sight, and making sure Chris hadn't following us, I said to Rob, "Don't worry mate, we'll get our own back on her, the miserable old cow" and we did but not in the way I had imagined.

On another occasion and attempting to carry on with the Ninja theme, we decided to blow up a bridge which crossed a small stream in the forest. I say bridge but in reality, it was nothing more than two strips of wood totalling eighteen inches wide and three feet long, but to us it was the 'Bridge on the River Kwai' and we were the assassins sent to destroy it. I'd pinched one of those jumbo-sized cans of hairspray from my mum and lighting a fire on the middle of the bridge, threw it on and we both stepped back about five feet.

"Nothing's happening," said Rob after about twenty seconds and I was just about to walk back over to the fire when... BOOOOOM!!!

The fucking thing blew up big style and even formed one of those ball of flames you see in the films. Pieces of twigs and branches came raining down on us and I remember thinking how lucky we were that no bits of the can hit us. It took a while for the smoke to clear and imagining the bridge to be history, we were both disappointed to discover it had only been scorched by the explosion.

"I thought you said it was gonna be like the 'Bridge on the River Kwai' said Rob, wiping bits of wood off his shoulders.

"Bigger!" I replied.

"What?"

"We need a much bigger explosion and next time, it should be underneath the bridge"

BIPOLAR.....MAYBE?
(Volume Two)

"How are we gonna make it bigger?" asked Rob.
"Next time we'll get some Bangers to add to the fire and you need to nick some hairspray off your mum too"
So that's exactly what we did but still the bleedin' bridge remained undamaged and yet it wasn't all bad news because when buying the Bangers, we also purchased a rocket that left us skint, 'so it must be good,' we thought.

Crouching down in the forest, about one hundred feet away from Chris's parent's house (they were away on their boat again) we stuck the rocket into the ground and angled it in such a way that it was directly pointed at the front door. Robert then scrambled up the slope and stood by the door waiting for my signal as I lit the fuse, and just as the rocket was about to go off, I gave him a wave. Rob then rang the doorbell and ran off down the lane and I waited for the rocket to take flight… and waited, and waited, and waited.

"The fucking thing has gone out!" I said to myself and could then see Chris opening the door.

He looked around for a couple of seconds and after not seeing anyone, closed the door again just before the rocket took off like… well, a rocket and smashed right in the centre of the door.

"Shit!" I said to myself, "That could have killed him!" and wondered what we were trying to achieve in the first place.

I suppose it never occurred to me that the rocket might actually hit it's target and was so relieved Chris had shut the door just in time.

"Fuck off you two!" he yelled after opening the door again and I wondered why me and Robert were doing these things to him.

Chris was our mate after all and I think it was just the fact he was alone in the cottage and we were bored out of our heads that we did these stupid things.

So that was it, me and Rob decided not to pick on Chris anymore but there was still the need to get even with his girlfriend, yet that revenge was not to occur until Christmas Eve, a couple of years later.

We'd been to a nightclub in Ilford and I was so drunk that at one point, I sat on a chair that had a tray full of glasses on it and smashed the lot without noticing. I honestly can't remember the name of Chris's girlfriend but she was there with him, along with myself, Robert and Ed. The girlfriend had arranged with her mum to pick us up at the end of the night and as we all staggered out of the club, there she was waiting for us. Chris, his girlfriend, Robert and Ed all squeezed onto the back seat and I sat in the front alongside the mum and was definitely feeling the worse for wear. I'm never sick when I just drink lager but, on this occasion, and still being relatively young, I was necking shorts back like there was no tomorrow. About half an hour into the journey, it was decided that I would be dropped off first because I was the nearest, but the motion of the car, combined with the alcohol I'd consumed, was starting to make me feel sick. When the car unexpectedly went over a bump, I suddenly vomited without warning and the sick sprayed all over the inside of the windscreen and bounced back not only over me but also over the girlfriend's mum.

"Open the window! Open the window!" she yelled, and winding it down, I stuck my head outside.

BIPOLAR…..MAYBE?
(Volume Two)

Exactly at that moment, a group of drunken revellers were staggering along the pavement singing, "Merry Christmas everyone!" and I could feel myself starting to be sick again.

You've heard of the expression 'projectile vomiting,' well that's what came spurting out of my mouth and it covered this group of people, causing them to fall silent in an instant, before realising what had happened.

"And a Merry Christmas to you too!" I thought to myself.

"You fucking cunt!" I heard faintly as the car carried on, and everyone on the back seat shouted and screamed at me for filling their nostrils with such a noxious odour.

Luckily (for me anyway) I felt a lot better when I was dropped off shortly afterwards and Chris rang me on Boxing Day to say that his girlfriend had spent most of the hours of Christmas morning, cleaning all the sick out of the car. So, like I said earlier, I got my own back but it definitely wasn't planned.

Justice!

A couple of weeks later and into the new year, me, Rob, Simon and Ed went to this pub in Chigwell which we'd never been to before and at some point, me and Rob shared a spliff in the car park and couldn't stop laughing at the smallest of things. Once back inside the pub, we carried on laughing, but neither me nor Rob noticed that Ed was getting pissed off with us (probably because he wasn't in on the joke, which in our condition could have been absolutely anything) At one point, Robert said that he needed some fresh air and I went outside to the car park with him again, but we failed to notice that Ed and Simon had followed us this time. Ed was still holding his half-filled pint of lager and when Robert started to feel better, he began laughing again, which set me off too.

"Are you fucking laughing at me?!" yelled Ed to Robert, but Rob didn't have a clue what he was going on about and then started to laugh even more than last time.

Ed then put his glass down on the bonnet of a car, went right up to Rob and stared straight at his face.

"I'm talking to you!" he said in a threatening tone and then for no reason at all, headbutted Rob and punched him twice in the face in quick succession.

This caused Robert to fall down to the ground and Simon went over to him to see if he was okay. Blood was pouring from his nose and it was lucky he didn't break it, while Simon, being the sort of person who would always have a clean handkerchief on him, held it under Rob's nose to stem the flow of blood. Personally, I've never seen the need for a handkerchief… that's what your sleeves are for ain't it.

"What the fuck are you doing?!" I shouted at Ed, "Leave him alone!"

"You fucking keep out of it!" yelled Ed and picked his glass up before smashing it on the bonnet of the car and holding under my chin, "Unless you want some an' all!"

I'm usually an extremely cautious person and constantly have my wits about me, but the effects of the spliff must have clouded my judgement and I failed to act (meaning, get out of his way quickly)

BIPOLAR.....MAYBE?
(Volume Two)

I could actually feel the cold of the glass pressing against my skin and immediately knew I mustn't do anything to antagonise him any further, because anyone who is willing to cut someone with a broken glass (friend or not) has got a serious problem controlling their anger and shouldn't be given a reason to go ahead with his threat.

"Whoa... forget about it," I said in the calmest voice I could muster and told myself I would never fully trust him again.

Much to my relief, Ed threw the glass away and then him and Simon went back inside and I helped Rob to his feet and told him to come back with me (my mum and dad's house was only a mile away)

When we got there, I sneaked Rob upstairs without anyone noticing and helped to clean up his bloodied face in the bathroom.

"I'll kill that cunt," said Robert once we were in my bedroom and I gave him a cigarette but had to steady his hand to light it.

I could tell he was shaking with rage and told Rob about not trusting Ed anymore, and although we all remained friends, both me and Robert remained wary of him in the future and said we'd watch each other's backs.

PART THREE: RECREATION

CHAPTER 27

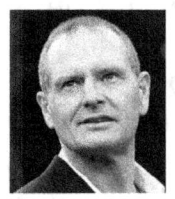

1985
Me, Robert, Ed and Jerrod started getting into the habit of gate-crashing private parties just for a laugh and would usually try houses where the front door was on the latch. These parties were much easier to sneak into because we didn't have to knock on the door or ring the bell and once inside, it was just a matter of mingling in with other people. That was the only thing we didn't have any control over, because the people at these parties could be completely different to us and on those occasions, our ruse was discovered relatively quickly. One such party was on the top floor of a small set of flats and was almost next door to the pub we had been drinking in. The main door to the building had a security lock however, so it meant hanging about until someone either left the block of flats or entered it. We then had to rush to the door without being spotted before it closed again and obligingly, a couple went inside just after we had arrived. Following the sound of the music, we climbed the stairs to the top floor and again our luck was in because the door to the flat wasn't locked. Once inside, we smiled and nodded at people as we worked our way to the kitchen in search of the booze

BIPOLAR.....MAYBE?
(Volume Two)

supply, which in this case was rather plentiful. Listening to all the people talking made me realise we didn't fit in at all because they were really posh and once we had grabbed a couple of cans each, we walked through the living room and out onto the balcony. It was absolutely packed with revellers, which was a good thing in a way because we stood over by the balcony and tried not to be noticed, but it wasn't long before this bloke came up to me and started up a conversation.

"How do you know Jeffrey and Pippa?" he asked while lighting up a cigarette.

"Well, erm…"

"I'm sorry, how rude of me," he interrupted and offered me one of his cigarettes.

"Don't mind if I do," I replied and after he had lit it for me, I tried to walk away before he could strike up the conversation again.

"So how do you know them?" he asked again while placing a hand on my shoulder.

"Oh well I… er," I mumbled and looked over to Rob, Jerrod and Ed, but they quickly turned their heads away and pretended to be in deep conversation.

"I er… well my sister actually… she was friends with Pippa at school and…"

"Oh, your sister is here too?"

"Well, no… she couldn't make it so I'm here instead"

"So, you're friends with Pippa too?"

"Yes, but erm… when I was a little kid"

"I don't know her myself," explained this bloke, "It's my girlfriend who is friends with Pippa"

"Oh right," I said, "anyway, I better be going…"

"Could you point her out to me?"

PART THREE: RECREATION

"Eh?"

"Pippa... could you point her out to me? I can't find my girlfriend anywhere and would like to introduce myself"

"Oh... yeh, she's er... that girl over there," I replied and pointed to this young woman stepping out onto the balcony through the patio door.

"The girl in the red dress?"

"Yes... and the blonde hair. Anyway... I'll leave you to it..."

Much to my horror, the girl in the red dress started to walk over in our direction and the man held onto my arm.

"Sarah," he said, "this is... I'm sorry, I didn't catch your name"

"Er... it's Jack," I answered and was confused that he was introducing this girl to me, instead of the other way round.

"Jack... this is Sarah," he replied, "and this is our apartment and our party"

"But what about Pippa and what's his name?"

"I have never heard of a Jeffrey or Pippa before and it is clearly obvious that you and your friends are gate-crashing!"

"Ah... well... I suppose then that we'd better be leaving..."

"Leave? Yes, and if you don't, I shall have you all thrown out!"

To be honest, this bloke remained really calm throughout our confrontation and my mates must have heard the whole thing because they started following me out of the flat without any prompting.

BIPOLAR…..MAYBE?
(Volume Two)

"And you can put those cans of lager down as well," said Sarah in the red dress, and we all walked out of the party with our tails firmly between our legs.

On another occasion, it was just me and Ed looking for a party to crash, and finding ourselves in Chigwell, we made our way to where all the big posh houses were. It was a lovely summer's evening and we could hear loud music coming from nearby and turning the next corner, a group of people could be seen drinking in the front garden of this house.

"Don't let them see us," explained Ed, "we'll go in once they have gone back inside"

"But what if they don't go?" I asked, as we hid behind some conifers of a front garden, a few houses down.

"They're gonna want to get another drink at some point," said Ed and as if right on cue, all these people walked back into the house and left the front door wide open.

As soon as they'd disappeared inside, we ran up to the house before casually walking to the door, inside the hallway and directly towards the kitchen. For all the houses me and my mates gate-crashed, if we at least got one sip of a drink before being thrown out, it was deemed as a success. The kitchen was packed with people laughing and drinking and luckily, we were able to open a couple of cans of beer without being questioned. As time went on, we found that nobody seemed to realise we shouldn't be there and our confidence started to grow until we walked into the living room where the music was playing and started talking to a couple of girls.

PART THREE: RECREATION

"I need to go to the toilet," I explained to Ed after about half an hour.

"There's a bathroom at the top of the stairs," said one of the girls, "the downstairs toilet is blocked up with sick"

She painted such a pretty picture and telling Ed I wouldn't be long, I started to make my way up the stairs. The bathroom was full up with people and seeing two blokes using the toilet at the same time, I looked over to the bath to see it was being used as a kind of giant urinal, with four blokes lined up side by side and pissing into it. When the end person had finished, they zipped up their flies and left and so I took his place and pissed to my heart's content.

"Alright John… I didn't know you knew Greg," came this voice to my left and turning my head, I saw my brother Davey pissing at the other end of the bath.

"Alright Dave," I said and then mouthed silently, "I don't"

Davey nodded his head and realised I shouldn't be there and after finishing his business, he turned to walk out the bathroom and said that he'd see me later. In one way it was good that Davey spoke to me because at least I now knew the name of the person who's house it was (well, his mum and dad's house, who were clearly not there) and making my way back downstairs, I got myself another can of beer from the kitchen. There was no sign of Ed, so I realised he must be in the living room and walking through the doorway, I saw him snogging one of the girls we had been talking to. I knew there was no chance of me getting off with someone 'cos the other girl was nowhere to be seen, and so I went back into the kitchen, necked my beer in one go and grabbed another one.

"That's my lager you're drinking," came this voice behind me and turning round, I was faced with this angry looking bloke and two of his friends.

"Sorry mate," I replied, "I must have taken the wrong one"

"Too right you did," he said, "where's your friend?"

"Er... I think he's in the other room... why?"

"Cos the both of you haven't been invited, that's why"

"But I'm here with my brother... he's friends with Greg"

"Alright then, if he's mates with Greg, show me where your brother is"

Scanning the kitchen, I couldn't see Davey anywhere and said he must be in the living room.

"After you," said this fella and him and his friends then followed me into the other room.

"Well?"

I couldn't see Davey anywhere and guessing he must have already left, explained it to this bloke.

"I saw a couple of people leaving about five minutes ago," said this girl, "two boys"

"So, you came here with your brother but he's left without you?"

"Well, I'm a big boy now and can go out all on my own," I replied.

"Here Greg!" called out this fella, and someone I vaguely recognised came over to us.

"Alright Pete, what's the problem?" he asked.

"This bloke says he and his mate came here with his brother... do you know him?"

"Nope, never seen him before. What's the name of your brother?"
"Davey... er... Dave"
"That's a common name... Dave who?"
I really didn't want to give out our surname but realising I didn't have any choice, I replied, "Barrett"
"Oh, so you're Dave's brother. Now you come to mention it, I have seen you before"
"So, everything's okay?" said the other bloke.
"Yeh, no problem but he's gone without you"
"That's okay... I'm here with a friend," I explained and pointed over to Ed who had his tongue stuck down this girl's throat.
"That's my girlfriend!" said the man who questioned me in the kitchen and marching towards them, pulled Ed away from her.
"What the fuck do you think you're doing?!" yelled Ed and pushed the bloke across the room, causing him to crash into a table full of drinks.
Now, I'm not someone who usually likes fighting but seeing as Ed was outnumbered by about fifty-to-one, I leapt towards this group of blokes who were about to grab hold of Ed, and started punching them on their backs.
"What ya doing you idiot!?" shouted Ed, "Hit them in the face!" and as if to give me a lesson, he swung a fist at the nearest fella, which made contact with his chin and knocked him to the floor.
It was at that point everything became a bit of a blur and fists and feet were flying everywhere as we were slowly pushed out of the house, with punches raining down on us. Eventually, we found ourselves back

outside and waiting to get our breath back, we then rang the doorbell, not really expecting it to open but a short while later, this girl let us in and we headed straight for the kitchen. Before even reaching the kitchen however, we were spotted again but me and Ed had promised ourselves that we'd at least get a drink inside us before being ejected from the premises again. So, with a group of about eight blokes trying to drag us back out again, we somehow managed to struggle forwards and pick up two cans of lager that had already been opened. Don't ask me how but we were each able to get a sip of beer as fists rained down upon us and it took these blokes about ten minutes to get us out of the house again because we gave as good as we got.

Once finally back out in the front garden (again) Greg came to the door and told us to fuck off and just before he slammed the front door shut, I yelled out that Davey wasn't really my brother and he was just a friend of a friend.

Walking back down the street nursing our wounds, I eventually said to Ed, "Well… what are we gonna do now?"

"I don't know about you," he replied, "but I'm going home"

"Are you sure?" I answered, "There's supposed to be this other party going on a few streets away"

"Fuck off!"

PART THREE: RECREATION

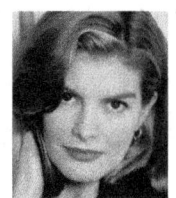

CHAPTER 28

1998
Although I wasn't what you might call happy working at Simon's place, the plus side of it was I didn't have the pressures of the family business anymore (see Volume One) and that had a positive effect on me and Debbie's marriage. Whereas I bottled everything up before, I was now able to talk freely with my wife and after the kids had gone to bed, we would stay up until two or three o'clock in the morning, just talking about anything and everything. There couldn't have been a more marked difference in my behaviour and those times were really nice (although bleedin' knackering when you had to start work at eight o'clock the following morning)

We started going to nightclubs again every other weekend and on the Saturday evenings we stayed at home, we still had a really good time. Looking back now, it seems so obvious that I was suffering from bipolar because if we were talking about someone we hadn't seen for ages, I would then get up at about seven o'clock on the Sunday morning and go and visit them without any warning. I was wide awake and just assumed everybody else to be the same, but as you

can imagine, not everyone was pleased to see me at such an hour and would say, "Bleedin' hell John... do you know what time it is?"
They would still let me in though and we'd talk for ages, with me rabbiting on and on, and them sitting there still dressed in their pyjamas and not being able to get a word in edgeways. Just thinking about it now makes me feel kind of embarrassed but hey ho, what's done is done. I've mentioned it numerous times before but when I start going high, things begin to spiral out of control and it always ends badly. For instance, when I said that me and Debbie were really on good terms, it was perfectly true and yet my erratic actions would eventually harm our relationship in one way or another.

1999
I had started getting into the girl group 'All Saints' after hearing their song 'Never Ever' which I thought was a great song and still do. It's one of those songs I think will really stand the test of time and on hearing that alone, I bought the album on the strength of it.
There was me earlier in the book going on about boy bands and girl bands and how little I thought of them, but to me, 'All Saints' were different and had this kind of maturity about them that other girl groups lacked (Spice Girls and the like)
I though it was great that they did a cover of the Red Hot Chili Peppers song 'Under the Bridge' and their version of 'Lady Marmalade' was really good too but I also liked some of their other stuff like 'I know Where It's At'
It's funny now though because I don't think I would

ever want to listen to that album again, but 'Never Ever' is still a really good song and it's great to hear it when it's sometimes played on the radio. People who know me would be quite surprised at my liking 'All Saints' because I was more into Blues and Rock music at the time, and nothing else would do. I suppose my tastes started to widen at the onset of House Music, which I immediately fell in love with, and from there my tastes became broader and broader, although I have to say, the Blues will always be my favourite and my love for it has never wavered (especially when I'm on a bipolar low, although love wouldn't seem to be the right description when I feeling that way)

Anyway, I'm going a bit round the houses here because I wanted to start writing about the time me and Debbie went to see the 'All Saints' at a gig in Shepherds Bush Empire on the first Saturday in May and we dropped the kids off at her mum and dad's 'cos they were going to spend the night there. It was a bank holiday weekend and I can always remember the weather being really nice, so we thought we'd make a day of it and have our lunch at a restaurant in Notting Hill. Well, that was the idea but it didn't go quite to plan because upon our arrival at Shepherds Bush Station, we decided that we'd go to a bar first and have a drink. We found a great little pub on the opposite side of the green to the venue and I noticed on a blackboard outside, that they were selling two bottles of Becks for the price of one. So, we sat down outside and seeing as I had two beers in front of me, it was only fair that Debbie had two glasses of wine and as time started to pass, the idea of having lunch became a distant memory. Because we could see The

BIPOLAR…..MAYBE?
(Volume Two)

Empire on the other side of the green, we could also see when a queue started to form outside, but this must have been about eight hours later and we had been drinking all that time, without any food inside us. When the queue eventually started moving inside, we stood up and that's when I knew I'd had far too much to drink but wanted to hide it from Debbie because she seemed absolutely fine. As we walked towards The Empire, I struggled not to sway all over the place but must have managed it because Debbie didn't say anything and once inside, I thought I'd order another beer before the gig started (stupidly thinking this would make me feel better)

Moving away from the bar, we pushed our way through the crowd until we were about fifty feet from the stage and right at that moment, the group came on. They opened with the song 'Bootie Call' (I only know this because I've just looked up their setlist for the gig) and I don't think I even made it until the end of the song before collapsing to the floor. I have no recollection of the next twenty minutes or so but Debbie told me afterwards that two security staff members carried me through the crowd and into the first aid room, which was positioned just off a corridor to the right.

The next thing I remember was waking up on this rubber type bed thing with Debbie looking down at me and when I wiped my mouth, I could see sick on my hand.

"Are you alright?" she asked quietly.

"Er… yeh… what happened?"

"You collapsed about thirty seconds into the first song"

"Oh"

PART THREE: RECREATION

"They're still on now if you want to go back and see them"

Propping myself up on my elbows, I looked down at my Tee-shirt and could see that was covered in sick as well. "I don't think I should," I mumbled and noticed this man standing next to Debbie who I guessed was the first aid person for the event.

"He'll be okay," he said to Debbie, "just had too much to drink that's all"

I sat up and swung my legs off the side of the bed and that's when I noticed all these teenage girls, who must only have been twelve or thirteen, staring at me with horrified expressions on their faces. I guessed that they were big fans of the 'All Saints' and when they finally got to see their heroines in the flesh, they fainted out of pure excitement. The same couldn't be said of me however and I was just this drunken slob who must have looked like an old man to them. Debbie appeared to be really embarrassed and who could have blamed her, I was feeling the same myself and just wanted to get out of the building as soon as possible.

Reaching the entrance of The Empire meant working our way back through the crowd again and I could feel all these eyes on me as if to say, "There's that idiot who can't handle his drink"

The group were still performing up on the stage but they were the last thing I wanted to look at and when we finally made it outside, I made Debbie promise not to tell anyone. As we made the train journey home, I suddenly felt really hungry (owing to the fact I hadn't eaten since the previous day and had puked up anything left inside of me) so when we got back home, we

BIPOLAR.....MAYBE?
(Volume Two)

ordered a Chinese takeaway and I scoffed myself silly before crashing out on the sofa.

When we went to pick the boys up from Debbie's mum and dad's the next morning, I lied to Ron and said it was a really good day/night and fair play to Debbie because she booked two more tickets for my birthday to see them again at Wembley Arena at the end of the year, and this time I made sure I ate something before going on to the booze.

So, the moral of that little story is, don't get paralytic drunk on an empty stomach and especially when you're going to be in the presence of a load of teenage girls!

PART THREE: RECREATION

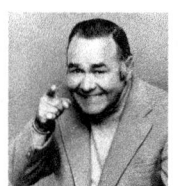

CHAPTER 29

Talking of gigs, me and Debbie would go to see loads of groups and solo artists and she was really good at getting seats close to the stage. I remember us going to see the Kinks at the Town and Country Club in Kentish Town on the August of 1989 and she was pregnant with our eldest son. It was a really good venue without any seating and was pretty small, meaning everyone had a good view of the stage and we managed to work our way right up to the front. The only thing with this meant it could get quite rowdy, with people pushing and shoving each other, and what with Debbie being pregnant, I had to place each of my hands on the stage, either side of her so she wouldn't get pushed about. Because of this, when the Kinks finally came on, Debbie got to shake Ray Davis's hand, which was great for her (lucky cow) and at a point in the show, Kirsty MacColl came on stage and performed 'Days' with the band (she'd just had a hit with their song)

Debbie's dad was into his music too and would often come along with us and although he was obviously older than me, I introduced him to a lot of bands that were closer to his era than mine. At the time, I was a massive Pink Floyd fan (I still like them a lot but not as

BIPOLAR…..MAYBE?
(Volume Two)

obsessed as I used to be) and me and Debbie had already seen them three times when she booked tickets for me and Ron to see them at Earl's Court in October 1994. The band would always open with the first five parts of 'Shine On You Crazy Diamond' with its distinctive fade-in of a G minor chord, played on the keyboard by Richard Wright. This time however, I thought they had made a variation to it because I could hear what sounded like a rumbling of thunder (just the sort of thing they would do) and less than a minute later, all the house lights came on in the arena. Me and Ron were situated on the side seating (on the left if viewed from the stage) and turning my head to face the back of the arena, I could see that the stand holding 1200 people, had collapsed to the ground. If you've never been to Earl's Court, you have to imagine that the seating is probably twice as high as a house and it's a miracle no one was killed, with bodies trapped in the scaffolding around them. 96 people were injured however, with 36 needing hospital treatment but none of the injuries were really serious and the concert was re-scheduled for a couple of weeks later. As spectacular as the Floyd gigs were, the musicianship was still of an extremely high standard and if you like guitar like me, then you can't go wrong with Dave Gilmour. Sadly, Richard Wright passed away in 2008 and although it's a shame not being able to see the band play live anymore, it was the right decision not to perform without him because his 'sound' was an integral part of the band's style. Of course, Roger Waters played a major part in Pink Floyd's writing, with a great deal of his lyrics becoming almost legendary and my only regret is not seeing him play live with the rest of the group because he quit in 1983. I did see him perform 'The Wall' live at the O2 arena in the Millennium Dome in 2011 however (man, I've listened to that album so many times) so that was kind of the next best thing.

Anyway, that's enough about Pink Floyd and my preferred concerts now are those with the least amount of theatrical flair and fancy lighting, such as Jeff Beck's gigs that are just raw performances and mostly instrumental (when the music is that good, who needs words?)

I'm a big fan of Alvin Lee from 'Ten Years After' fame (who? I hear you ask) and after already seeing him with the band, me and Ron went to see his Albert Hall gig in May 2004. Ron was really suffering badly with a damaged knee at the time and struggled to even walk to the venue from the station, but once we were sat in the second row from the front (thanks to Debbie again) he didn't seem too bad. Now this proves the power music can have on someone because when Alvin Lee started to play (along with a drummer and double-bass player and no one else) Ron was in his absolute element (as was I) with the last thirty minutes of the gig being a rock and roll medley with lightning-fast guitar playing. Everyone was standing, apart from Ron because of his knee and when I turned to look at him at one point, I could just about hear him saying, "Marvellous! Bloody Marvellous!" and he had a massive smile on his face.

Out of all the gigs I've been to over the years, I can honestly say that was my favourite, with just three people on stage giving it their all. After the gig was

BIPOLAR…..MAYBE?
(Volume Two)

over, we had the same walk back to the station, but this time Ron was striding along and didn't once mention his bad knee. Now that's the effect music can have and in the words of the late, great Alvin Lee, "Rock and Roll never dies!"

Two other great guitarists I saw (four times each) were Gary Moore and Jeff Healey, both of whom having also died far too early and at one of Gary Moore's gigs, Albert Collins came on stage and it was so cool seeing them play off one another. At the end of the concert, George Harrison also came on and that was a real surprise because at that point in his career, he hardly ever performed live. At around this time, Eric Clapton was doing an 18-night residency at the Albert Hall and if I remember correctly, this was his third year in a row. Because he has had such a long career, the gigs were split up into three parts, with the first part being his more pop orientated songs, the second part devoted to Blues and the final part being accompanied by a symphonic orchestra. Debbie booked the tickets again but chose the first, pop themed gig and although he's a great guitarist, I was gutted not to see his Blues nights on stage.

I suppose the worst gig I ever saw was Status Quo at Wembley Arena because you could tell they just didn't have any enthusiasm and didn't really want to be there. Don't get me wrong, I know their guitar playing is not in the same league as those I've previously mentioned and to me, they are almost like a guilty pleasure, but when they said, "What shall we do next?" and started playing the theme to the Batman TV show, I knew I didn't want to be there either.

PART THREE: RECREATION

Me and Debbie went to see Aerosmith (also at Wembley Arena) but I don't remember much because I got pissed, only that it was rumoured they might not perform because Steve Tyler had laryngitis (blimey, how he screamed out those songs I'll never know)
Talking of rumours, we went to see Fleetwood Mac but again I was disappointed because Lindsey Buckingham had just quit the band and that was the only reason I wanted to see them in the first place. My cousin Mick always said I was born in the wrong era because of my love for all these bands from the late 60's and I only wish I had been old enough to see Peter Green's version of Fleetwood Mac, oh… and a bit of Hendrix too, that wouldn't have gone a miss either!

Capital Radio starting doing these gigs called 'Party in the Park' during the late 90's and early 00's and Debbie booked for me and her to go to Hyde Park on the July of 1999. Capital was a really popular London radio station (I don't know if it still is 'cos I don't live there anymore) and so the concerts were attended by over 100,000 people, meaning the atmosphere was really good, even if half the crowd were kids who had gone along with their mums and dads. Although I would have avoided many of the acts like the plague, there were some groups I was keen on seeing, such as Eurythmics, Madness, Blondie and Elvis Costello. The ones I could have easily missed included Geri Halliwell, Martine McCutcheon and Boyzone and although I wasn't a fan of Culture Club, I was pleasantly surprised that Boy George's voice sounded exactly the same as on their studio recordings. Ricky Martin was pretty good (my

BIPOLAR…..MAYBE?
(Volume Two)

mate John would have loved that!) but to be honest, I was more interested in the female dancers than his actual singing. The weather was gloriously sunny all day long, which made it a lot easier to put up with the rubbish performers who I had expected to be crap, but there were still loads more who were even crapper (Thomas) too.

Anyway, the whole experience couldn't have been that bad because we decided to go again the following year and this time we took our eldest son with us, who would have been ten at the time. It's good when you see someone who surprises you and Bon Jovi was one of those groups, with the whole band sounding as professional as the acts I mentioned earlier but if I'm honest, they're not really my cup of tea (too middle of the road soft rock for my liking)

I was surprised how well Christina Aguilera sang, but this was quite early in her career and she later went on to prove just what good voice she has. All Saints were there but my enthusiasm had started to wane a bit by then and I can hardly remember much about them at all. Bryan Adams was pretty good (still a bit soft for me though) and Destiny's Child were very good, as to be expected, but still not really to my tastes. There was the usual crap again, including Victoria Beckham (I really don't know how she had the nerve to perform on the same stage as Beyoncé) Melanie C and Billie Piper. Suggs came on stage but without Madness this time and although he hasn't got the best voice in the world, I bet you he wouldn't deny that fact and think he was singing to the standards of some of the other acts. It just goes to show what a difference the weather makes though

PART THREE: RECREATION

because after about four hours, it started to rain and instead of drying up, the rain got heavier and heavier and, in the end, we decided to leave. Missing the rest of the concert did mean however that we failed to see the likes of Queen, Elton John and Marti Pellow so, it wasn't so bad after all because I would have really struggled to watch that lot.

On the whole though, I've been pretty lucky with the gigs I've been to, mainly because the bands performing had been around for years and really knew how to play live.

Sorry if that part of the book went on a bit and who really wants to know what gigs I've been to? I can't really explain but I sort of needed to get those things written down because they played such a major part of my life with Debbie and anyway, I could have told you about the many, many more we went to see, so think yourself lucky!

CHAPTER 30

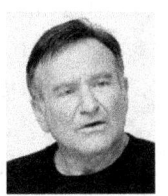

October 2001

Our daughter Leonie was born at the beginning of July (she was the only one of my kids I never saw being born 'cos I didn't get to the hospital in time) and although we were obviously feeling very happy, it was becoming increasingly obvious that the area we lived in was rapidly going downhill. About a year earlier, this family had moved in directly opposite us and while I got on well enough with the dad, his two sons were a bleedin' nightmare (was my own childhood coming back to haunt me?) and they would run over the tops of parked cars and all that sort of stuff. I reckon the eldest of the two was about ten years old but it was the younger son, who must have been six or seven, who was the real pain in the arse. Anyway, I'd been suggesting (vigorously) to Debbie that we should think about moving to a better area and she finally agreed and acknowledged our street just wasn't what it used to be. We found a house for sale about three miles away and although that wasn't very far, the properties there were considerably more expensive, as was reflected in the general attitude of the people living there. We knew this to be true because Debbie's friend lived in one of the houses and she told

PART THREE: RECREATION

her what the area was like. So, we put our house up for sale and on this particular Saturday afternoon, a couple were due to come round to view it. We'd had a big extension built on the place several years earlier and even if I say so myself, the house was really nice (which explained Debbie's initial reluctance to move)

Whereas it was a four-bedroom property, the house we wanted to buy only had three bedrooms and the kitchen was tiny compared to the one we already had, but as I said, the area was much nicer and so this was reflected in the price. I got to view the house before Debbie and the idea was also to have an extension on this place, so I took a tape measure and pen and paper with me and took the relevant measurements in order for us to do just that. Debbie told me we should get the place even before she had a chance to look at it herself because by now, she had her heart set on it and knew the layout of the houses anyway because of her friend's place.

Being as the house we were trying to sell was ex-council, the price was governed by that, but they were lovely little homes (well, ours wasn't little anymore) and built just after the war. The three-bedroom house we were after had been built in 1932 and were private instead of council, and when one of them came up for sale, they would always go really quickly, hence Debbie's eagerness to get things moving as quickly as possible.

The couple coming to view our house were due at two o'clock and about ten minutes beforehand, I kept looking out of the living room window, to see if they had arrived yet. The dad of the family I just mentioned was about my age and talking to him in the street a

BIPOLAR…..MAYBE?
(Volume Two)

couple of days earlier, he explained that his own dad was seriously ill in hospital and things didn't look good. Being as our house was an end of terrace property and therefore the final house at the end of the street, we were literally less than a minute's walk away from our two boy's school, which was situated opposite our road on the street running perpendicular to it.

"They're still not here yet!" I called out to Debbie who was in the kitchen.

"It's only just gone ten to," she replied, "come away from the window… it won't make them get here any sooner"

"Maybe they've changed their minds and aren't coming. I knew something like this was going to happen!"

"It's not two o'clock yet and keep your voice down, you'll wake Leonie up"

Nin was asleep upstairs in her cot and Debbie was putting the kettle on, in case the viewers wanted a cup of tea.

"Where's Sean and Robert?" I asked, "It's very quiet upstairs"

"They've gone round to their friends," said Debbie, "you should know, you were supposed to be keeping an eye on them"

Looking out of the window again, I saw the youngest of the two kids from opposite, climbing over the school gates before crouching down and getting something out of his jacket pocket.

"What's that little brat up to?" I asked myself and then saw him get a lighter out of his pocket and set fire to what I guessed was some paper and sticks.

PART THREE: RECREATION

When the fire was underway, he removed some more sticks from his pockets and added them to it before going over to one of the bins and emptying that on the fire too.

"Fuck it!" I said out loud as the flames started to get bigger and bigger.

"What was that?" asked Debbie.

"That fucking kid from over the road has just lit a fire in the school playground!"

"How do you know?"

"Cos I'm looking straight at him... the little git!"

"Do you think the people coming to look at the house will notice?"

"I'd be surprised if they didn't, you can see right through the fence"

"What are we going to do?" said Debbie as she walked into the living room, "It might put them off"

"He's climbing back over the gates now," I replied, "I'll go and speak to him"

"Mind what you say... you know what he's like, he'll probably end up throwing a stone at our window or something"

Debbie was absolutely right because that's exactly the sort of thing he would have done if I had started having a go at him, and as I opened the front door and stepped outside, he came running over from the other street and headed towards his house.

"Oi... kid!" I called out (well, I didn't know what his bleedin' name was did I) "Come over here for a second!"

"What for?" he replied and had a look on his face that you really wanted to punch.

BIPOLAR…..MAYBE?
(Volume Two)

Walking over to him and trying not to look angry, I stooped down and said, "Your grandad's not very well, is he?"

The boy didn't reply but looked at me in such a way that said, "How does he know about that?"

"Your dad has got enough on his plate as it is," I continued, "and the last thing he needs right now is the aggravation of you starting fires in the school playground"

I was about to say if he went and put it out straight away, then I wouldn't say anything to his dad but I didn't have to. I've never seen a kid run so fast as he raced across the street, climbed back over the gates and started jumping up and down on the fire until it went out. I then went back inside and looking out of the window again, saw him making his way back to his house and going inside. Just as he shut the front door, a car pulled up outside our place and it was the couple who'd come for the viewing. I think this couple actually ended up buying the house but I can't remember for sure and we moved into the other place just before Christmas.

Because the house needed new windows (they were the original ones and let the cold draft in terrible) and there was no carpet on the ground floor but exposed floorboards instead, the place was freezing and what with the tiny kitchen and bathroom, we went through the process of getting planning permission for the extension as soon as possible. The whole thing went relatively smoothly, apart from having to dig the footings an extra metre deep (which I mentioned earlier) although by the end I swore we would never do

PART THREE: RECREATION

it again and the work on the house was completed in just over a year. Out of all the homes on the estate, I reckon ours had by far the biggest driveway and it was possible to park up to eight cars on it, so by the time the boys had learned to drive and had their own cars, we still had plenty of space when people came to visit.

It's funny because when me and Debbie eventually split up, it was my decision to leave because I just didn't want the kids seeing us argue anymore and I always remember her saying, "But what about all the work you've done on the place"

"That don't mean a thing Debbie," I replied, "it's not the house you live in but the things that go on inside that really counts"

CHAPTER 31

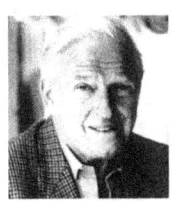

Going back to the American bloke called Ross who spoke to me when I was digging the footings. We did as he suggested and went for a drink in the Cricketer's pub a couple of days later and really hit it off. What I liked about Ross was that he wasn't your typical competitive American who bragged about them being the best country in the world and how they were better at everything than anybody else. Far from it, he was a massive fan of the UK and especially admired Winston Churchill, who happened to be a member for the parliamentary constituency of Woodford (where I lived) from 1924 to 1945 and then up to his retirement after the war. That was the main reason Ross chose to live in the area and at the top of our street was (and still is) a statue of Churchill which made me feel proud every time I went passed it.

When the extension to the house had just started, I had to cut door sized holes in some of the walls with an angle grinder (the fucking dust was a nightmare, I tell you) and then carry the bricks out to a skip on the drive. My two boys had recently bought some really cool BB guns (before they were banned) that looked just like a pair of real 1911 Colts and along with the kids next door who also had some guns, they were involved in a shoutout, where my boys were firing from the upstairs bedroom window. These other kids were hiding behind a parked car in the street and as I carried the bricks to the skip, pellets were flying all over the place, bouncing off lamp posts, cars and even me. It was a really sunny day and as Ross crossed the street and walked onto the drive, I warned him about the pellets and told him to watch out. Just at that moment, a pellet narrowly missed his head and bounced off the skip we were standing next to.

"Fuck me... this is just like being back in Nam!" he yelled jokingly while grabbing my arm, "Let's take cover inside!"

I reckon Ross was about eighteen years older than me and really had done a tour of duty in Vietnam, and over the years I knew him, he told me some really harrowing stories.

I made a point of not asking him about the war but after we had been to the Cricketer's three or four times, he began to open up about it and explained the time he got back to America at the age of nineteen after being in Vietnam for a year. The plane flew into Washington, DC from Saigon but instead of a pre-arranged connecting flight to Boston Logan Airport (Ross lived in Massachusetts with his parents at the time) he had to call them and ask for the plane fare to be wired over so he could organise a flight himself. His parents willingly obliged but seeing as it was a commercial flight and once on board, Ross quickly realised he was the only passenger in uniform and even at that young age, knew exactly what a large percentage of the American public thought about the war in Vietnam.

"I was sat next to this old guy," Ross told to me, "but looking back, I'm guessing he must have been in his forties"

Ross then went on to explain that the man must have been on a business trip because he was wearing a suit and had put a briefcase in the overhead locker. About twenty minutes into the flight and looking at a magazine someone had left behind in the seat pocket in front of him, Ross saw out of the corner of his eye that the man next to him pressed the button above his head to call for an air hostess. When she arrived a short while later, the man whispered something in her ear before the hostess walked away to the front of the plane. The man then started to look up the aisle every few seconds and five minutes later, he stood up and made his way to the front of the plane after grabbing his briefcase. Curious as to what he was doing, Ross slid across into the now vacant seat and leaning over to see what was going on, he noticed the man sitting down in a seat further up the plane. It now became obvious to Ross that the man didn't want to sit next to 'this kid in a uniform' but at least he now had an empty seat next to him and could stretch out a bit more.

Once landed in Boston and after exiting the plane, the passengers showed their passports and then waited to collect their luggage on the baggage carousel. Ross quickly found his rucksack and was about to leave the airport when he noticed the man in the suit waiting for his own luggage, a little further along. Walking up and standing behind him, he then tapped the man on the shoulder and waited for him to turn around.

PART THREE: RECREATION

"Then what happened?" I asked Ross, eager to know the outcome of the story.

"John," replied Ross, "I hit that man harder than I'd ever hit someone before in my life and walked away.

"That's great!" I said laughing, "I wonder what happened to him?"

"As I was walking away, I turned round and saw the guy unconscious, going slowly round on the conveyer belt"

"Did security say anything to you?"

"Back then, security was much more lax and nothing like today. Nobody stopped me and I walked straight out of the airport, got in a cab and made my way home"

Once back home and after several weeks trying to live like a 'normal' civilian, Ross got a job working in the offices of a local paper as a file clerk, and most of his days consisted of going from desk to desk, giving letters and paperwork to all the different employees. A television in the main office was constantly tuned to a news channel with the sound turned down and on this particular day, Ross happened to glance over at it and read the headline which stated a gunman had opened fire on innocent people at a nearby shopping mall. Someone else turned the volume up and all the employees stopped what they were doing and turned their attention to the TV screen. When details of the casualties were announced, Ross suddenly dropped the paperwork he was carrying and hid under a desk and refused to come out for several hours. Not wanting to explain his actions to his superiors, he never returned to the company again and instead got a job working in a

BIPOLAR.....MAYBE?
(Volume Two)

'Gas station'

By this stage, Ross started using Smack and as the months passed by at the gas station, his addiction grew and grew until he found himself in desperate need for more cash. At home, he started stealing money and jewellery from his family and was also rapidly turning into an alcoholic, and after months and months of trying to get him clean, his parents finally had enough and threw him out.

The owner of the gas station began to trust Ross and as time went by, he allowed him to live in a storeroom out the back (it sounds like the Steve Martin film The Jerk) and as the trust grew and grew, the boss gave him a set of keys and would let him open up the business in the mornings. In the owner's office inside the gas station was a safe where he kept all the takings from cash transactions and although Ross liked him a great deal, the temptation to steal the money to feed his addiction was too great. He'd previously spied on his boss and saw him punch in the combination to open the safe and one night when alone, Ross opened it up and helped himself to the contents which amounted to roughly $5000. Being as he'd known the gas station owner kept the money in the safe until the Friday and would then take it home to put in the bank the next day, Ross stole the cash on the Thursday night, realising the total would be at its greatest before the following day.

At this point, Ross contacted his parents and they allowed him to return home but he would be supervised when he was around any of their valuables. The $5000 went within a couple of weeks and in total and utter despair, Ross didn't know what he was going to do, but

PART THREE: RECREATION

his parents then received a phone call a couple of days later, with someone official asking to speak to their son. Basically, it was an authorised call explaining to Ross that the government had just introduced a system to fund a benefit scheme for all U.S veterans, where they would receive a fixed sum of money each month if they were unable to work. Along with this, a generous pension was also offered to each veteran and now finding himself in a comfortable position, Ross finally managed to clean his act up. In order to achieve this, he started paying regular visits to a psychiatric hospital for Vietnam veterans, but instead of being admitted as a patient, he gave talks to the vets about his life of drugs and thefts and how it was never too late for them to change their lives around.

At about this time and with money no longer being an issue, Ross decided he would like to visit all the well-known war graves throughout Europe and that's when he settled on England as his base and when I first met him.

One of the patients in the hospital was this guy called Jim, who'd stay in his room and standing only a few inches away from the wall, would stare at it for hours on end. The doctors gradually allowed Ross to talk to him in his room and with both men being Vietnam veterans, Jim slowly began opening up to Ross and eventually joined the rest of the patients in the main hall. When Ross came to England the following year, he knocked on my door and had Jim with him and it just goes to show what faith the doctors had in Ross, by allowing Jim to accompany him. I did notice he was pretty quiet (compared to Ross anyway) but he seemed like a good person and I would meet up with them regularly at the Cricketers. Both of them visited Italy the following week (Ross fell in love with the place and now lives there with his Italian wife) and after touring the war graves and it was time to return to the U.K, they were actually permitted to board a U.S military aircraft and flew back to England free of charge.

On another of Ross's trips to the U.K and being your typical tourist, he decided to visit the Houses of Parliament and upon exiting the building via the main front door, he bumped into John Reid, who was the Secretary of State for Defence at the time. They spoke for a couple of minutes, with Ross explaining he had fought in Vietnam but obviously being a busy man, Reid finally said he had to go and started to enter the building.

"Just one more thing," called out Ross before Reid disappeared.

"Yes… what is it?"

"You seem like a really nice man but you treat your veterans like shit"

Ross said that Reid nodded slightly in agreement before disappearing out of sight and realised he must have known about the benefit scheme operating in the U.S.

PART THREE: RECREATION

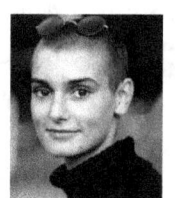

CHAPTER 32

It was during the summer and I was working in the kitchen of the house in Pilgrim's Hatch (the one with the snake, the frog and the pipistrelle bat) when my mobile rang and it was Ross on the other end of the imaginary line.
"Hiya Ross, how you doing mate?" I asked.
"Hi John, you need to come round tonight at say... half seven"
"Why, what's up?"
"Oh, there's nothing wrong... far from it in fact," he replied and sounded in a very good mood.
"Can't you give us a clue?"
"Nope, it would spoil the surprise... only that it's wonderful. I'll see you later," he answered and with that, he ended the phone call.
"Wonderful... what could be wonderful?" I asked myself and for the rest of the day, I tried to figure out what this 'surprise' could be, with the possibilities growing and growing until I became convinced Ross was a secret millionaire and was going to give me loads of money.
"I can't wait to see him," I told myself and worked away happily until five o'clock.

BIPOLAR…..MAYBE?
(Volume Two)

Driving back to my place, I was already thinking how to spend my new found wealth and couldn't wait until half seven arrived.

I was having my dinner after I got home, when my phone beeped and it was a message from Ross.

"Ask Paul if he wants to come along as well," it read and my heart sank a little because it meant Paul was going to get a share of the lolly that was rightfully mine.

"Okay," I messaged back and then rang Paul (my friend who I went to the Catweazle convention with in Volume One) and told him about Ross's cryptic call.

"I'll meet you outside your flat at 7:15," I wrote and he agreed on the time.

So, meeting Paul at the designated time, we walked the fifteen-minute journey to where Ross was staying and he answered the door upon ringing the bell.

"Hey John… hey Paul!" he said with a big smile on his face and stood to one side so we could enter the house.

I'd been there a couple of times before after Ross kept saying what a great place it was and he was absolutely right; it was almost like stepping back in time which appealed to my nostalgic sensibilities.

By the look of it, I'm guessing the house was built in the 1800's and had two large bay windows on either side of the porch, which had those black and white tiles on the floor, resembling a chess board. The place was (and still is I hope) owned by this lovely couple called Penny and Martin who were I'd say, in their late fifties at the time. The garage was to the left of the house and stood unattached, with the doors open to reveal an old Austin Morris with the bonnet propped open. I guessed Martin must have been working on it because there were spanners and such lying on a bench next to the car and knowing the type of person he was, it didn't surprise me at all.

Penny was an English tutor at a nearby university and Martin was a mechanical engineer who could turn his hand to most things (hence working on the car) which always ended up with perfect results. It was almost as if they'd turned their backs on the modern world, with one of those old Bakelite telephones sitting on a small wooden table by the kitchen door and there wasn't a television to be seen anywhere. What appeared to be original antique walnut furniture filled the rooms, none of which were in that great a condition, but instead had the look of cabinets and tables that had been used frequently over the years. They did in fact own a television, but it looked pretty old and was concealed underneath a detailed patterned cotton tablecloth and sat on the top of a waist high cupboard.

"Where's this surprise then?" I asked in jest, as all three of us stood in the hallway.

"Ah… you'll just have to wait until eight o'clock," replied Ross and led us into the living room where Penny and Martin were seated.

Both of them were reading books when we entered the room and although they had met me before, they had never seen Paul and so Ross introduced him to them. After about ten minutes of conversation (much of which went right over my head but Paul seemed to know what they were going on about) I asked Penny if it was okay if Ross showed Paul his bed (an unusual request I grant you) and she said of course, it was Ross's room anyway, for the duration of his stay with them. Martin

BIPOLAR…..MAYBE?
(Volume Two)

had built an extra bedroom in the loft space, complete with an en-suite bathroom and there was also a hinged window which you could walk out of, onto a small balcony that overlooked miles and miles of rolling scenery as far as the eye could see.

As I mentioned earlier, Ross used to rent a room in the house opposite to mine and Debbie's place but he had a bit of a falling out with the husband of the place (he was I bit of an arsehole I admit) and found Penny and Martin's place after being introduced to them by Winston Churchill's former secretary (I told you he was a big fan) This lady also lived close to us and although by now very elderly, Ross said she still had all of her faculties and invited him over for tea one time.

"So, Winston actually came to visit you here?" he said after taking a seat.

"Laddie," she replied, "you're sitting in his chair!"

It turned out that for most of his time while working, Churchill opted to spend his time at his secretary's home because she was far more organised than him and always knew exactly where to find a relevant file or document, should it be required. To most people it would sound far fetched when Ross came out with these stories (he also introduced me to this brilliant magician) but being the type of person he was, he would start talking to absolutely anyone and because he had such a friendly way about him, those people in turn would become his friends.

Penny and Martin's house was a much nicer place to stay at and before I ever went there, Ross told me that he slept in this great room with a terrific view, and it even contained a Jacobean four-poster bed. I took his

PART THREE: RECREATION

comment with a pinch of salt however, believing him to be exaggerating... that is until I saw the bed for myself. Upon setting his eyes it, Paul was as gobsmacked as I had been because it really was this great big four-poster bed with intricate designs of men and women involved in sensual acts carved into each of the wooden post. That sounds a bit tacky but I can assure you the carvings were very discreet and they somehow fitted in with the whole design perfectly.

"Surely it's a reproduction?" said Paul (which was exactly my first response) and Ross then went on to say that Martin had made it himself.

The fucking thing was huge and made from dark oak, with two dark red velvet curtains tied back on either side of the headboard, which was also this great big piece of oak. It really was a thing of beauty and must have taken ages for Martin to complete... blimey, was there anything this man couldn't do? Judging by the size of it (each post must have been at least ten inches in diameter) I reckon the whole thing weighed more than a ton and I just hope he built it in such a way that it could be dismantled, otherwise if they ever decided to move, the bed would have to have been incorporated into the sale of the house.

I'm supposed to be the woodwork instructor where I work now, which is a bleedin' joke because if I had made it, the thing would have been constructed out of old pallets with rusty nails sticking out of it!

(I'm a right old bodger sometimes)

"We've got to go downstairs now... it's almost eight o'clock," said Ross, interupting Paul who was closely inspecting the beds carvings.

BIPOLAR.....MAYBE?
(Volume Two)

"What do you think it is?" mouthed Paul as we followed Ross into the garden.

Three deckchairs had been erected in a semi-circle and in front of them sat a radio on top of a small round garden table.

Looking at his watch, Ross then said, "I won't keep you in suspense any longer," as we all sat down on the red and white striped deckchairs, that looked like they had seen better days.

"Well?" I replied.

"There's a documentary on Radio Two all about Laurel and Hardy and it's just about to start now," he responded while leaning forward and turning on the radio.

Like me and Paul, Ross too was a big fan of Laurel and Hardy and don't get me wrong, I do love them but I was expecting to be rich beyond my wildest dreams and did my best to conceal my disappointment (I'm only joking of course... well, sort of)

It actually turned out to be a really good night; a lovely summer's evening with plenty to drink (I made sure of that by bringing my own personal supply) and after the documentary, we must have talked and talked until about midnight, with the conversation concerning all things film and old TV shows (right up my street)

"So much for being millionaires," I said to Paul as we walked home and thinking about it now, that was the last time the three of us saw each other together again.

After my diagnosis with bipolar and eventually moving down to Hampshire to live with my mum and dad, Ross came to stay for a couple of days, but my dad had died by then, although he did meet him before, when me and

PART THREE: RECREATION

Debbie lived in Woodford and we had some friends round. Although the visit from Ross was nice (I had taken some time off work) it wasn't quite the same somehow, maybe because I was wondering what he thought of me after knowing I had a mental health condition. In hindsight, I realise that train of though is utterly ridiculous because if anyone knows about mental health problems, it's my good friend Ross.

CHAPTER 33

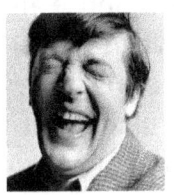

Saturday, 13th May 2006

The second I woke up; I knew I was in a really good mood but seemingly for no apparent reason.

By now, all of the work on the house was complete (maybe that was something to do with it) and me and Debbie were due to go to my uncle Johnnie and aunt Sandra's joint 60th birthday celebration later that evening. They were actually born in the same block of flats on the same day and their births were assisted by the same midwife. Little did they know they'd end up getting married and would spend the rest of their lives together.

Debbie was still in bed when I got up and so I made a cup of tea and took it up to her (blimey, if ever I needed a sign something was wrong, that was it!) and because the weather was good, I decided to cut the grass. By now, the kids had woken up and were watching TV and by the time I'd finished the grass, Debbie had started doing some ironing (ours and not her customers) and so I decided to clean the cars.

You know you get one of those days when you are full of energy, well, I was certainly feeling like that and as I was finishing off the cars, my neighbour had come out

PART THREE: RECREATION

the front and started talking to me. I ended up going into his house and speaking to him and his wife (I've no idea what about) and can always remember the exact date because West Ham were playing Liverpool in the Cup Final and it was showing on their TV. I probably spent an hour round there and when I finally walked back into my own house, Debbie asked where I had been because my car was still there. I think she was a bit fed up with me (no change there then) and always acted a bit strange when it came to the neighbours because she hardly ever spoke to them on either side of us. I must admit, I've never liked to get too close to a neighbour because it can end up with you having no privacy and having them constantly knocking on your door, but that certainly didn't apply to those particular neighbours. I wish I could remember their names because they were a really nice couple and although the wife was English, her husband was Greek but you would have never known it because of his London accent.

About an hour after I had got back indoors, Debbie's mum and dad turned up because they were taking the kids back to their place for the night and when they eventually left, I had a shower and shave and started to get ready. A minibus had been arranged to take us to the party in the West End and when it pulled up outside at half six, me and Debbie climbed aboard and were greeted by my mum and dad, my eldest sister Pauline and her husband Dave, my sister Ellie and her husband at the time called Bob, and my brother Davey and his partner Helen. Since then, Davey and Helen have married but I warned him not to rush into anything because they had only been with each other for twenty

BIPOLAR…..MAYBE?
(Volume Two)

years! Oh, and there was the driver too, a bloke named Bert who had a gammy leg and a glass eye and could speak twelve different languages (not really, I just made that bit up, although for all I knew, he could have spoken twelve different languages… I mean, something like that would have come in handy being a minibus driver) and even though he appeared to be a decent enough chap, he could in fact have turned out to be a serial killer or something.

Anyway, my mum and dad, Pauline and Dave and Ellie and Bob had driven up from Hampshire earlier in the day and my mum and dad were staying at Davey and Helen's, while the others had booked two hotel rooms for the night. I've already mentioned that the party was in the West End but unfortunately, I can't remember where exactly and although I could ask Pauline or one of the others, I'm too ashamed after what happened later that night and don't want to remind them of it. The journey took just under an hour because of the traffic (even on a Saturday) and looking back on it now, I was absolutely 100% experiencing a bipolar high, although no one knew it at the time (including myself) and I didn't stop talking at a hundred miles an hour for the whole way there.

The minibus dropped us off on the edge of a plaza which was surrounded by upmarket jewellers and high-end clothes shops and I remember there being some bronze statues on display as we neared the end of the square and turned into a narrow street housing a fancy looking Italian restaurant. Johnny has always loved his Italian food and does a lot of business over there and as a consequence, has many Italian friends. Upon entering

PART THREE: RECREATION

the restaurant, a man took our coats and hung them up (not that I was wearing one 'cos it was a warm evening) and we were each then offered a glass of champagne from a waitress carrying a silver tray. Over to the left and up a couple of steps was a dancefloor and ahead of us and up a few more steps was where all the other guests were. Johnny and Sandra greeted us all and then we helped ourselves to the tasty nosh on display and chatted with all our cousins and uncles and aunts.

A couple of hours later, music could be heard coming from the direction of the dancefloor and after smoking a cigarette outside, I joined Debbie and we began dancing with some other people. I never ever saw my dad dance in all the years I knew him and so it came as no surprise that he was propped up at the bar with my uncle Tommy, who also never danced. Saying my dad was propped up at the bar makes him sound like an old boozer but nothing could have been further from the truth. The only time he ever really drank was when he went to Portugal a couple of times a year with my mum but being surrounded by her family in this restaurant made him feel awkward and so he drank to try and relieve that feeling.

I on the other hand, do like a drink but only lager and never spirits and my dad had always said to me and Davey that people who drink in the daytime will never amount to anything in their lives and would end up with nothing. Those words of wisdom must have had some effect on me because I never drink during the day and only after nine o'clock at night. It's just a little rule I have and I've always stuck to it. Anyway, because me and Debbie were spending so much time on the dancefloor, I didn't really have time to drink much and as a result, I remained relatively sober for the rest of the evening (that's important to mention because of what happens later that night)

At one point, I went for another cigarette and walking back into the restaurant, I got a drink for Debbie and myself (only one of a few I can assure you) and whilst waiting at the bar, I looked over at my dad and could see had had one of those spiteful looks on his face that I could remember vividly from my childhood. He was staring directly at my mum who was by now also enjoying herself on the dancefloor and the expression in his eyes said, "Look at her, fucking enjoying herself!"

It sounds absolutely ridiculous because what was wrong with her enjoying herself, and yet that's exactly how he could be; almost as if he were jealous in some way but couldn't do anything about it. My uncle Tommy was still standing at the bar and I got talking to him for a while and during this point, my mum came off the dancefloor to get herself a drink. Even though I was in conversation with my uncle, I could overhear my dad swearing in hushed tones to my mum and so she walked off and went back to the dancefloor again. She didn't even wait to get her drink so along with mine and Debbie's, I took hers too and gave it to her.

Even though I was having a good time, I kept staring over towards my dad and could see that fucking nasty look on his face that I had grown to hate so much. Trying not to let it get to me, I started to dance with Debbie again, while my mum and her sister Maureen (Tommy's wife) were in hysterics at something or

PART THREE: RECREATION

other. Again, I went for a cigarette and then back to the bar to get a drink for Debbie (I was drinking slowly for some reason and didn't want one) and this time, my dad was talking to Tommy and they were both effing and blinding about Maureen and my mum having such a good time without them.

"Listen you pair of cunts," I whispered to them, "this isn't about you two… it's their brother's birthday and they are enjoying themselves"

Oh man, I should have realised there was something not quite right with me because I would never have spoken to them in that way usually. Needing to calm myself down, I went back outside for another cigarette and Tommy came out to join me.

"You're a sensible man John," he said, "and you're right"

"I'm sorry Tom," I replied, "I shouldn't have spoken to you like that"

"No… you were right to. Me and your dad can be miserable fuckers and it needed saying"

I nodded my head and finishing the cigarette, walked back inside and got myself a beer.

"Don't you ever fucking talk to me like that again," said my dad in my ear but I just shook my head and joined everyone back on the dancefloor.

At midnight, the party was still going strong and I could tell my mum wasn't letting my dad's mood get to her, because she couldn't stop laughing as she carried on dancing. A short while later, Ellie's husband Bob said that we'd better start leaving because the minibus had been booked to take us home at half twelve, but looking over towards my mum, I could tell she wanted to stay

BIPOLAR…..MAYBE?
(Volume Two)

and so I told Bob that I'd go and tell the driver to wait.
"But it's booked for half twelve," he repeated.
"That's alright," I replied, "we'll give him an extra fifty quid… he'll wait for that. Give us a tenner towards it"
Begrudgingly, Bob put his hand in his pocket and gave me the ten pounds and then I asked my brother to do the same. I then went to Pauline's husband Dave to ask for a tenner and as he gave it to me, I thought he was going to have a heart attack, judging by the expression on his face.

At that point, Debbie came over and said, "Pauline's saying are we ready to go? It's still early yet"
"Don't worry," I replied and explained the situation before stepping outside and making my way to where the minibus had dropped us off earlier.

The driver didn't look too happy at my request, but when I showed him the fifty quid, his eyes lit up and he said, "No problem"

Walking back to the restaurant, I was surprised that all our group (apart from my mum) were standing outside and my brother said they all wanted to go home. I looked at Debbie who just shrugged her shoulders and Pauline then went inside to fetch my mum.

Half an hour later, we were driving back on the A12 and I was sat in a single seat behind the driver, with my brother up front beside him. My mum and dad were sat behind me, Debbie was seated next to Helen on the other side of the minibus and behind them were Pauline and Dave, while Ellie and Bob sat right at the back. At one point, I briefly turned round and saw my mum silently gazing out of the window with a smile on her face and I could tell she had really enjoyed herself and hadn't wanted to leave so early. I was experiencing a really weird sensation that I don't recall ever having before, and that was my mind seemed to be racing at a million miles an hour and my senses appeared to be razor sharp. For example, and because I was sat alone and wasn't engaged in conversation, I could hear everybody else on the minibus and what they were all saying at the same time. Well, that's the way it seemed to me at the time, but now I know a great deal more about the effects bipolar can have on the mind, I realise it was a case of me being extremely alert to all the things happening around me and what was being said. Of course, being directly behind me, the things my dad was saying to my mum were much more prominent and so when he said, "I'm sorry Pat," it was almost as if he was talking straight into my ear.

"Give it a rest will you dad," I said to him while turning my head to face him.

Normally, I wouldn't have said anything but I'd heard it so many times on previous occasions, I just got fed up with hearing the same thing over and over again and knew thay were just empty words.

"Don't you fucking talk to me like that, you little fucker!" he growled back and that's when things went a little off kilter, to put it mildly.

"Mother fucking cunt!" I yelled while turning around and grabbing hold of his shirt collar.

Everyone else on the minibus fell silent (at least I think they did 'cos I couldn't hear them over the noise of me and my dad screaming at each other) and my dad then grabbed my shirt and pulled me closer to him. We then started exchanging blows and I've got to laugh because my mum just sat there in silence, bemused by what was happening.

"You cunt!" I shouted.

"You fucker!" yelled my dad.

"I'll kill you… you fucker!"

Ellie's Bob must be about six foot four and sitting at the back of the minibus, he stood up and leaned forward in an attempt to calm me down.

"Sit down John!" he said, "We're in a speeding vehicle!"

"You fucking sit down!" I yelled, "Or I'll fucking bury you!"

God knows what the expression looked like on my face, but I'm guessing it was pretty threatening because Bob sat down in an instant and remained silent for the rest of the journey.

The A12 is a dual carriageway that's about eight or nine miles long and widens into three lanes at certain points but has no hard shoulder. Because of this, the driver was unable to stop the minibus and instead of slowing down, he accelerated even harder, I'm guessing so he could get off the road as soon as possible. Thinking about it, he was surprisingly calm, but I guess he'd seen it all plenty of times before while taking drunken people home; the only difference this time being that I wasn't drunk.

Finally, we made it to the Green Man roundabout in Leytonstone and taking the exit that headed towards Woodford (where we lived) the driver was able to pull over into a bus stop. All the while, me and my dad were still fighting and Pauline yelled over the racket, "They can walk home from here driver!"

PART THREE: RECREATION

Her words must have registered in my mind because I immediately stopped attacking my dad and Helen then called out to my brother up front, "You go with them David"

Helen always speaks really well (not like I does) and Davey climbed out of the minibus and opened the side door. Debbie got out in an instant and I followed her while my dad kept saying, "My boys... where are my boys going?"

I wasn't fooled by his words however; he may have cared about Davey but he didn't give a fuck about me and once I was stood on the pavement, I leaned back into the minibus and grabbed hold of his legs. Pulling as hard as I could, my dad slid out of his chair and across the floor towards the open door while my mum held onto his wrists and tried to pull him back. It's as if he was some kind of human Christmas cracker, but instead of revealing a gift, a stream of obscenities spewed out of his mouth.

Helen then leant forward so she was staring out of the open door and told me to, "Stop!" and with that one word, I immediately let go.

Thinking back now, it's funny because as soon as I did stop, the door slid shut and the minibus wheel spinned away before I had a chance carry on trying to hit my dad.

I suppose it must be three miles from where we were dropped off to our house, and as we walked back, my brother remained about thirty feet in front of us all the way.

"Why doesn't Davey want to walk with us?" I asked Debbie.

BIPOLAR…..MAYBE?
(Volume Two)

"He's scared of you," she whispered and I noticed that she too kept some distance between us.

I couldn't believe what she said to me because there was no way I would do anything to harm Davey and I was just about to say something to him when Debbie grabbed my arm and shook her head.

"Oh well, that was an eventful evening!" I said out loud in an attempt to lighten the mood but no one laughed and I decided to keep my trap shut.

It took about 45 minutes to get back home and once there, Debbie ordered a taxi for Davey and he stood outside until it arrived, so maybe there was some truth in what she said to me. As soon as he had gone, Debbie went to bed without saying goodnight and so I went in the kitchen, grabbed a beer from the fridge and stepped out into the back garden to light a cigarette. Inhaling the smoke deep into my lungs, I then let it slowly escape from my mouth and said out loud to an empty garden, "Oh fuck it!"

PART THREE: RECREATION

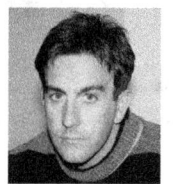

CHAPTER 34

It was eleven o'clock the following morning and there was a knock on the door. Debbie had hardly spoken to me since we'd woke up a couple of hours earlier and upon opening the door, I was faced with my mum standing on the porch step. Looking over her shoulder, I could see my dad sitting in their car which was parked on the street and not on our drive, and I noticed him looking over in our direction.

"We're just on our way back home," said my mum, "can I come in for a minute"

"Of course you can," I replied and stepped to one side, "but not him"

Closing the front door, there followed a few seconds of awkward silence until my mum finally asked, "Why John, why?"

Not really having a sufficient answer, I just shrugged my shoulders in silence and then mumbled something about dad being drunk.

"It was a party," she answered, "everyone was drunk"

"John wasn't," said Debbie walking out of the living room, and that was the first thing she had really said since we had returned home the previous evening.

"I heard the way he spoke to you," I told my mum, "and

saw the way he was looking at you. He had that horrible expression on his face"

"Oh, come on John, you know what he's like when he gets drunk"

"That's no excuse… he's an ignorant pig and I never want him to set foot inside this house again"

"Don't talk about him like that"

"I mustn't talk like that about him, but it's okay for him to treat you the way he does?"

"He doesn't mean it and has apologised already"

"Like he always does and says he'll never do it again… until the next time. I heard him on the minibus"

"You shouldn't have behaved like that while we were driving along," said Debbie and I noticed she wasn't looking me in the eye as she spoke.

"I know," I replied, "that was wrong of me and I'm sorry… but I'm not sorry for hitting him"

"Well, if that's still the way you feel, there's no more to be said," answered my mum and giving me and Debbie a kiss and saying goodbye, she was gone.

As I shut the front door, I became aware that my ribs were hurting and as the day progressed and then back at work the following day, the pain was getting worse and worse until I eventually went to the hospital for an x-ray.

"You have three broken ribs," said the nurse holding two radiographs up to the window so I could see, "how did you manage to do that?"

I shrugged my shoulders and lied about being drunk, and then the nurse said I shouldn't do too much physical work for the next few weeks.

Even though me and my dad had that altercation on the

PART THREE: RECREATION

minibus, I still wasn't quite sure how I managed to break three ribs, until it suddenly dawned on me. It had to have been when my dad was pulling me towards him and I was being forced against the back of my chair, but even so, he really must have been pulling hard for that to happen.

When I got back to my car, I spent the next half an hour phoning all the others who had been on the minibus and apologised profusely for my stupid actions.

Two days later on the Wednesday, me and Debbie were making our way to the Albert Hall on the train to see Dave Gilmour (of Pink Floyd fame) in concert. Before we left home, I looked on his official website and it recommended a pub to visit which was close to the venue and upon arriving there, the place was absolutely buzzing and had a great atmosphere. It was down a cobbled mews and opposite the pub, I noticed an antique car dealership with three Ferraris on display.

"Do you reckon that place has a connection to Nick Mason?" I asked Debbie but she said she didn't know and we just enjoyed the company of the rest of the customers (most of whom I reckon, were also going to the gig) until it was time to start walking to the venue (oh, by the way… Nick Mason is the drummer from Pink Floyd, in case you were wondering, who's known for his huge collection of Ferraris)

Once we'd entered the Albert Hall and shown our tickets, I looked at my watch and told Debbie we had time for another drink in the bar, but as soon as we were given them, she kept saying we had to hurry up or we'd miss the beginning of the gig.

"We've still got twenty minutes," I told her, "and our

seats aren't that far anyway"

It's funny 'cos although I'd introduced Debbie to Pink Floyd, she was the one who was panicking and had become a big fan of Dave Gilmour herself.

"Come on John, hurry up!" she said while finishing her glass of wine and I had to down my pint off in a couple of gulps (you weren't allowed to take drinks into the show)

I was still feeling hyped up from the Saturday (and still didn't know why) and it was almost like I was purposely taking my time in an attempt to calm myself down (and was doing a pretty good job of it)

As Debbie started running to the auditorium door that led to our seats, I walked slowly as if I didn't have a care in the world and when my arse finally came into contact with the seat, the curtains came up and the band came on... perfect timing!

As to be expected, the gig was brilliant and included guests David Crosby and Graham Nash from Crosby, Stills & Nash, who performed on a couple of Dave Gilmour's recent songs. Seeing as she'd really enjoyed herself, Debbie seemed to open up to me a bit more, which was really the first time since the minibus incident, and walking back to the station after the gig, she kept saying how good it was. With my mind still finely tuned however, I was able to listen to what she was saying, while being completely aware of our surroundings, including what was going on behind us. Even though the pavement was busy with people making their way to the station, I could sense this bloke about ten feet away to our rear and don't ask me how, but I just knew he was following me and Debbie,

PART THREE: RECREATION

probably in the hope of mugging us or something, when things quietened down. Leaning over, I whispered in Debbie's ear about him but she just scoffed and said I was being paranoid. I do realise now that paranoia can be a symptom of bipolar disorder but I knew for sure I was right and so stopped in my tracks, knelt down and pretended to tie my shoelaces.

"What are you doing?" asked Debbie after walking on a couple of steps, and then returning to where I was knelt.

"Won't be a second," I replied and then indicated the man to her with my eyes as he passed us.

Just then, he also stopped and started tying his shoelaces too and so I stared directly into his eyes and he stared back.

"You're going to look away first," I told myself and after a few more seconds, he stood up and carried on walking.

"Now do you believe me?" I said to Debbie when the bloke was a good distance ahead of us.

"It was strange, I must admit," she answered and when I stood up, we began walking again, but I told her to slow down.

"He might be waiting for us in an alleyway," I explained, "and could have a knife on him"

I could still tell Debbie wasn't 100% convinced about my suspicions but she did slow down somewhat and we never saw the man again.

When we were on the train going home, Debbie asked me if I was feeling alright and that I seemed on edge, but all I could do was shrug my shoulders and reply, "Yeah... I'm fine"

BIPOLAR…..MAYBE?
(Volume Two)

All through the rest of the train journey and the walk home, I kept thinking about that man and how I knew for sure that he was planning to mug us.

On the following Saturday evening, we went round to my cousin Mick and his wife Pauline's house for a BBQ and my second cousins Lee and Michelle were there, along with a load of other people. Debbie spent most of the night talking to Pauline, while I mainly chatted with Lee and Michelle and at about half eleven, I looked over to where Debbie had been standing and realised she wasn't there anymore.

"Have you seen Debbie?" I asked Michelle and she told me that she'd gone inside with Pauline.

Thinking no more about it, I carried on drinking and talking to Lee, when Mick came up to me and said that Debbie was upset.

"Where is she?" I asked.

Mick pointed towards the open patio doors and replied, "In the living room… Pauline's comforting her"

"What's up with her then?" said Lee and after shaking my head, I told him about the incident on the minibus on the previous Saturday night, believing that to be the reason.

This was confirmed when Pauline finally came outside and whispered to me that Debbie was upset because she had never seen me like that before and didn't realise I could act so aggressively.

I realised then that it was Debbie who had been scared of me that night and not my brother after all… he had been disgusted with my behaviour and didn't want anything to do with me.

"So, what's she crying about?" said Lee looking

PART THREE: RECREATION

genuinely confused, "She's married to a Barrett and should be used to it by now"

Pauline went back inside with two glasses of wine (and drank them both! Only joking) and after about another half an hour, Debbie walked outside into the garden. I asked her if she was okay, and she nodded her head in silence and then explained that Pauline had told her not to be afraid because, "John is a good man and would never hurt you. Those bloody Barretts have so many issues going back years and you have to realise that not all families are the same"

This was a reference to Debbie's dad Ron who was such a nice bloke and although he went through some bad times during rocky periods of his property business and started drinking heavily for a while, he was naturally a good person and a good dad and quickly got his act together again.

BIPOLAR…..MAYBE?
(Volume Two)

PART FOUR:
WOULD THAT IT WERE

PART FOUR: WOULD THAT IT WERE

CHAPTER 35

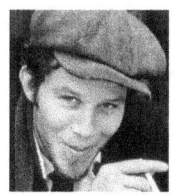

Would that it were... it doesn't have anything to do with this part of the book, I just like the sound of it, especially when Andrew Keir says it in Dracula: Prince of Darkness. Actually, thinking about it, would that it were might have some relevance here and there, so maybe it wasn't such an odd title after all.

In 'Volume One' I wrote about the possibility of Donald Trump becoming president and some of the ridiculous things he might get up to. He just so happened to be inaugurated into office on January 20th, 2017 and surprisingly enough, his presidency remained relatively uneventful (apart from his comment about drinking bleach to cure Covid or seemingly to encourage his supporters to march on Capitol, which many of them did, resulting in some deaths and interrupting the electoral vote count. He was the only American president to be impeached on two occasions and his meetings with North Korean leader Kim Jong-un proved to be nothing more than a publicity stunt, with no real progress on denuclearization being achieved. Although I wouldn't have voted for him if I'd been American, at least his time in power made the evening news a lot more entertaining, especially when compared to that of his successor Joe Biden, who looks like he's asleep half of the time, hence the nickname 'Sleepy Joe' from Mr. Trump.

Since 'Volume one' the entire world has been affected by the outbreak of Covid-19 and up until vaccines started becoming widely available, most countries were put under lockdown and even the pubs were shut (now, that is serious)

Thankfully, the vaccines started to make life return to normal to some extent but it's left the country heavily in debt, what with the furlough scheme offered to people unable to work in their usual jobs and certain members of the public who abused that system (you'll always get them)

The day service where I work all but shut down and if it wasn't for the domiciliary care we offer in some of our homes, I would now be out of work, much like my good friend Becks who was made redundant. Thanks to the vaccines, the day service opened up again last year and only up until recently, everyone (staff included) had to take a Covid test every single day, which was obviously a very good thing and gave many of our guys some peace of mind.

Then there was the debate about having the vaccine or not, with some people claiming it was a conspiracy and contained a drug that altered the mind to follow certain powerful individuals in their creation of a new world order.

"That's a load of crap," I told one member of staff who believed in all that stuff.

"No, it's not John, a leading doctor in the U.S has gone on record to say it's true"

"And where do you find out all of this information?" I asked her.
"On YouTube... where else?"
"Well... how about the news?"
"You don't want to believe what they tell you... it's all a pack of lies"
"How do you know that?"
"This psychologist on YouTube..."
And so on and so forth.
Some people thought it was a bioweapon created in a Chinese laboratory to wage war on America, others believed it was made as a plot to derail Donald Trump's re-election campaign and more still think it was caused by 5G mobile networks and once we were given the vaccine, a miniscule microchip was planted in our bodies and we then acted as slaves, brainwashed to serve some of the most powerful people in the world. These social media sites have become a breeding ground for like minded people and it's almost like Chinese whispers (created in a lab in China) where each telling of a particular theory, becomes more and more outlandish. I'm not sure if we'll ever know how the virus really came into existence but don't worry because we'll always have the conspiracy theorists to feed us with random bits of information. YouTube and Twitter and the like are all the same when it comes down to it, people are sharing information whether it be true or false but it doesn't really matter because there will always be people out there willing to believe anything. Many people, perhaps even the majority think the vaccine was created so quickly that the long-term side effects haven't been given the necessary time to

reveal themselves (that's if there are any) and I myself feel that way too to some extent, but I've still had the jabs and apart from having no hair, I appear to be just like any other ordinary member of the public. I honestly believe that the vaccine was created in such a record time because all the scientists and medical experts from around the world, dropped everything else so to speak, and concentrated their efforts solely on this one particular virus. That still doesn't excuse the fact that long term side effects haven't been properly recorded yet but hey ho, I (along with billions of other people) will just have to wait and see.

My mum was in Portugal when the lockdown was just about to commence and luckily, being able to change her flight, she ended up getting the last plane out of Faro before all commercial flights were grounded. Even though she loves Portugal and has many, many friends out there, she told me that she would much rather be stuck in England than another country. Some of her friends weren't so fortunate however and ended up being shut in apartments or hotels for months on end and after more than two years, my mum travelled back to Portugal once again and I could tell she was itching to do so because it's almost become like a second home. There were times during lockdown where it sometimes felt like a story out of a disaster movie, with empty streets and no traffic on the roads and I suppose that was the only real positive thing to come out of it. The main negative as far as I was concerned, was queuing up outside supermarkets, with only a limited amount of people allowed in the store at one time and even once inside, everybody had to follow the arrows and walk in the same direction. It was like paying a trip to Ikea every time I went food shopping but if that was the worst thing that happened to me, then I should consider myself very lucky. There were those poor people who died as a result of Covid, whilst others spent weeks and weeks in hospital, not to mention the nurses who looked after them all.

One of the very best things to happen during lockdown was of course Captain Sir Thomas Moore, who at the age of 99, walked lengths of his garden with the help of a walking frame and raised an astonishing thirty-two million pounds for NHS charities. He was knighted by the queen (who has since died and we now have a king... it still feels weird saying that) and Tom himself sadly passed away at the age of 100, which of course is a grand old age but it was still a shame even though it was expected. I think his story more than most, lifted people's spirits and showed that no matter how gloomy and depressing the news could be, there is always someone out there willing to make a difference, and he certainly did that.

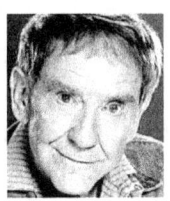

CHAPTER 36

Scrunched up sweet wrappers, chicken bones, used tea bags, banana skins, potato peelings, tin cans, rotten cabbage… sorry about that, I'm talking a load of rubbish! Speaking of rubbish, is it just me or are the drivers on the road getting worse and worse? See what I did there? See the link? Impressive eh!

This bad driving can range from either going too fast or way too slow, with all the stuff in-between being fucking useless and bleedin' dangerous. Say for instance that I'm waiting to turn right off of a main road into a smaller road but there is a line of traffic on the other side. Instead of leaving a gap, the driver will go up right behind the car in front, even though they're not going anywhere, making it impossible for me to turn and at the same time, causing a line of traffic to start forming behind me. To make matters even worse, for the most part they don't even realise they are doing it and have no awareness of anything else around them. It's the same when you are waiting to pull out of a road and they have nowhere to go, and yet still won't let you out. I know I'm going to get a load of abuse for this but nine times out of ten, it's a woman driver and you can see her with both hands clamped onto the steering wheel and she's gazing straight ahead, almost as if she's wearing blinkers. Men can be just as bad but in other ways because although they are usually aware of the traffic around them, they are arrogant as if they own the road and can be right behind you when you're driving along. It's times like that I wish I was driving a beat-up old Land Rover or something and quickly put my foot on the break, because they would crash their car right into the me and it would be completely their fault. By far the biggest issue I have however, is people who don't indicate and as the days go past, there seems to be more and more of them on the road. They disrupt the flow of traffic around them because the other drivers don't know what their intentions are but they don't care, just as long as they're going to get to their destination, and don't give a toss about anybody else. All this moaning makes it sound like I get all worked up (I don't use the word stressed because it is alien to me) but far from it, their useless driving amuses me in some ways and as long as they don't involve me in an accident, who cares. Another thing that really is alien to me is road rage and the idiots that get so worked up over the most trivial things. You'll see them blaring their horns and swearing out the window and for what? So they can ruin the rest of their day because they are in such an angry mood that they can't snap out of it and return to normality. They're just bonkers the lot of 'em and the language is fucking appalling! The only times I ever use the horn on my car are to either acknowledge someone I recognise walking along the pavement or to warn another driver that they're about to reverse into me or drive over a cliff and fall to their doom.

BIPOLAR…..MAYBE?
(Volume Two)

Although I left school without taking any qualifications (much to my detriment) I did learn one valuable lesson and that is to always show good manners in life and pay respect to those people who deserve it. I might speak a bit rough around the edges but I can't be accused of being impolite and it's something that I'm not only proud of, it also makes me happy because it's nice to be nice to others who deserve it and the ones that don't… well, I just don't bother speaking to them anymore and walk away (whilst whispering a merry tune to myself)
At school, we were taught to hold the door open for someone who is either behind you or coming in the other direction, and that is something I have always done. On one occasion, this woman seemed to take offence by it and said, "I am capable of opening a door you know!" and aside from thinking, "Oh shut up you silly old cow!" I replied, "I'm not holding the door open because you are a woman, I would have done it if you were a man, a boy, or a girl and it's the way I was brought up"
She looked at me as if I was mad and then stormed off, whispering some rubbish under her breath.
You then get people who don't appear to have any manners at all and will walk into a newsagent and say things like, "Give me a scratch card," or, "I want a packet of fags," without a please or thank you anywhere to be seen (or heard)
A lot of the younger generation seem to be lacking in these core values (I've definitely become a moany old git) and whereas my teachers and my parents taught me good manners, they don't appear to have been taught

PART FOUR: WOULD THAT IT WERE

anything at all... well, not in how to behave around others anyway.

In a forward at the beginning of 'Volume One' I wrote how certain individuals who have attended universities may be extremely well educated when it comes to the particular subjects they are studying but when it comes to everyday life, they can sometimes not even notice the bleedin' obvious, even if it's dangled right in front of them. A good example of this concerns my nephew who is super intelligent and has become a doctor after years of intense course work and training. He is definitely not one of those ignorant people with bad manners, but exactly the opposite and is a genuinely nice guy. He came round to my mum's house with my sister Ellie (his mum) and we were due to go out for a meal about half an hour later. During that time, we sat in the kitchen and talked over a cup of tea (or ten) and my mum mentioned how there had been a spate of burglaries in our area over the last couple of weeks, with someone attempting to break into the house next door. Anyway, when it was time to leave, me and my nephew (I know it should be my nephew and I but that's not how I speak and it would be misleading) walked out of the house and were about to get into his car. Ellie stood on the doorstep as my mum started to shut the front door but just before she did, she yelled out loud back into the house, "We won't be long John, see you soon!"

Both me and Ellie took no notice by my nephew started laughing and called out to my mum, "He's outside here with me nan!"

I rolled my eyes and explained that she was trying to make it look like someone would still be at home and

BIPOLAR…..MAYBE?
(Volume Two)

he looked at me with a surprised expression on his face and replied, "I would never have thought of that"
Bless his little cotton socks.

You know when you think you've written something before, well I'm sure I've already mentioned the contents of the last paragraph in one of my earlier books but I have scanned through them and can't see it anywhere. Just in case I have however, well… you're getting two for the price of one… or is that you're paying twice for the same thing? Oh, I don't bleedin' know, ask my nephew 'cos he's the educated one and will probably draw up a chart explaining the whole thing.

Oh yeh, I've just remembered something else concerning my nephew, but this time we were round Ellie's house (well, her old house to be exact because she now lives in Canada, which would be a long way to go, just to pop round for a cup of tea)

We were all sitting in the living room and 'The Searchers' was on the TV and it came to the point when Natalie Wood calls out the warning, "Unt meyer! Unt meyer!" meaning, "Go away! Go away!" I think.

(Forgive the spelling, it's supposed to be Indian (as in cowboys and Indians, which in turn should be known as Native American nowadays)

Oh, very quickly before I go on and of talking in a politically correct term, there was this woman on the BBC news reporting about the fishing rights dispute between Britain and France, and instead of saying 'fisherman' she actually said, 'fisherperson' and I couldn't believe me lug holes. Even the bloody spell-check on my laptop while I'm writing this, recognises fisherperson... what the fuck has happened to the world? Everyone is so scared of offending someone else, that they can't even say something that is in no way meant to be offensive!

Anyway, back to Natalie Wood. Just before she yelled out those words, I too called out, "Unt meyer! Unt meyer!" and my nephew looked at me and couldn't believe it.

"How the hell can you remember that?" he asked, "You must have seen this film hundreds of times!"

In truth, I've only seen 'The Searchers' about three or four times and explained that I can remember the most trivial things (usually film orientated) but when it comes to something of importance, my mind just goes blank. He on the other hand remembers things that really matter and that's why he will end up being wealthy and I'll just be a bum... a no-good loser, dirty bum! (and I'm not talking about an unwashed bottom)

I really hope it doesn't come across that I was being disrespectful to my nephew and others who are equally as intelligent, because that definitely is not my intention. I could never do what they have achieved in a million years and my hat goes off to them for studying so hard and for so long and in any case, they are having the last laugh because they probably earn about eight times what I earn and deserve every penny.

That reminds me and while we're on the subject of brainy people, I must ask my nephew a question that's bugged me ever since I was a little kid and that is:

If a boy (or girl or goldfish) is exactly ten years old (do goldfish live that long? Another question for him but I suppose I might as well look that one up on Google)

BIPOLAR…..MAYBE?
(Volume Two)

and his brother is exactly five years old, then the eldest boy is exactly twice as old as his brother. The following year however, when the youngest boy is six and his older brother is now eleven, the elder of the two is no longer exactly twice is age.

How the fuck does that work?

I bet Einstein or Stephen Hawking couldn't even figure that one out, even if they drew up all the charts in the world… or perhaps I should say universe!

PART FOUR: WOULD THAT IT WERE

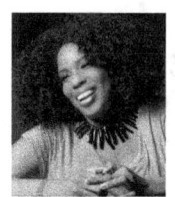

CHAPTER 37

What's with young blokes nowadays and skinny legs? In my day, men had proper legs like John Wayne, and they were even celebrated in that song 'John Wayne Is Big Leggy' by Haysi Fantayzee... that's how much real men's legs were regarded. It's not just their legs that are skinny, most of 'em look like they need a good dinner inside them, whilst conversely, girls have become fatter and fatter and seem to almost celebrate the fact, with blubber bulging out of ill-fitting clothing. There is a Frank Zappa and the Mothers of Invention album called 'We're Only in It for the Money' (love that album) and one of the songs on it is titled 'Take Your Clothes Off When You Dance' with a line saying, "There will come a time when you won't even be ashamed if you are fat" Now bearing in mind that album came out in 1968 and all the hippies at the time were probably stick thin, old Frank really hit the nail on the head and accurately predicted the future; more than he probably realised himself.

When I walk around Tesco doing the weekly shopping, in front of me will be a couple pushing their trolley along and while the husband might be made of nothing more than skin and bone, the wife is this grotesque slab of lard, wobbling her way down the aisle while throwing items into the trolley without a second thought or glance. There's a reason the husband is so thin, it's because he can't get a look in and the cupboards are bare before he has a chance to eat something. You then find you're stuck behind them at the checkout and before they've even paid for the shopping, the wife will be shoving a bar of chocolate or a cake into her gob and the checkout girl has no choice but to scan an empty wrapper. For fuck's sake, couldn't she have at least waited five more minutes until she was outside, before gorging herself?

I suppose I'm being a bit unfair (not to her, the greedy pig) because not everyone is like that, but I certainly remember the ones who are.

Whoops, I just remembered that my mate Becks did that very thing in 'Bipolar….. Definitely' but she's not fat… honest.

Another thing is the use of swearing being spoken so frequently nowadays and once again; I find that girls are worse than boys when uttering profanities. It's cunt this or fuck that every other word and although I'm no saint when it comes to swearing, surely there's a time and a place for such things and shouldn't be used in everyday conversation. It's as if the very fabric of a decent society has been gradually worn away and people just don't have the proper values, which I think are so important to living one's life, nowadays.

Nowadays, all you hear on the news or read in the papers, are incidents of people stabbing each other and on many of these occasions, the perpetrators are only kids of fourteen or fifteen years old. What the hell is

PART FOUR: WOULD THAT IT WERE

going on, don't they realise they're possibly (and frequently) taking another person's life? But the really worrying thing is that they do know the consequences of their actions and just don't care. It's cold-bloodied murder but to these kids, it's almost like having a badge of honour bestowed upon them and they are proud of the terrible crime they've committed. Why can't they stop and think about what they're doing before it's too late? That person they have killed will never be coming back, and there's nothing you can do to alter that fact! It's not a game or one of those crappy films starring one of those shitty actors... it's real life. Kids of my generation wouldn't have even considered killing someone in a million years, because such a terrible thing would not have entered their minds for even a split second and I must admit, hearing all that bad news on the TV makes me start to feel low and I sometimes struggle to snap out of it. But continue to watch the news I do because I think it's important to keep up to date with global events and I especially enjoy the goings on in the Houses of Parliament and all the shenanigans that goes with it.

There is that constant debate regarding censorship and the effects some films have on certain individuals, and I myself am of the belief we should be able to watch what we want, but only to a certain extent. There's a really fine line between what we should watch and what we shouldn't and who is it that makes those decisions? In this country it's the BBFC, who were famously known for banning movies they deemed unacceptable, but nowadays, things seem to have gone the other way and anything goes. The main issue has always been in

BIPOLAR…..MAYBE?
(Volume Two)

regards to horror films, with the 'video nasties' of the early eighties being a good example, but those movies seem like kid's stuff compared to some of the things being shown in cinemas in this day and age. These new horror films are just that, 'horrific' but not in the same way as a movie being scary or atmospheric used to be, and requires the audience to use their imagination at certain times during the film. The majority of today's horror movies are described as 'body horror' and for the most part, all they do is show images of extreme torture and mutilation. That's not a true horror film and all the makers have achieved, is to create a feeling of nausea and disgust amongst its viewers. Disgust that is, unless the member of the audience starts to enjoy what they are seeing and, in some cases, are even inspired by it. For the producers though, all that really matters are ticket sales and if the film happens to result in the death of a completely innocent member of the public, then so be it.

There will always be individuals defending such films of course, who say that any sane person with an ounce of intelligence wouldn't be influenced by what they are watching, but that in itself lies the problem because those defending these movies really are sane, rational people who assume everyone else is just like them. Let me say right now that not every person is of a similar state of mind, and it's these people who are too thick to differentiate between fact and fiction and truly believe it's okay to emulate the things they are seeing on the screen. It's not just movies in this day and age either, there are all those ultra-violent video games (is that the right term?) that may have been purchased by an adult, but are constantly played by kids as young as ten or eleven, once the adult has got fed up with it and tossed the game to one side. Don't get me wrong, I would have loved to have played those games myself when I was a kid but I promise you right now, I would never at any point have been influence to copy the things that were happening in front of me… even if I could have got my hands on a flame thrower or sub machine gun or even a bazooka!

Things were so much simpler when I was a kid and we didn't have the internet taking over our lives. It's now possible from the comfort of your home, to play such games with anyone, anywhere on the planet and the days of hide and seek and you're 'It,' seem like a distant memory.

Of course, we all had the school bully who made our lives a misery but, in my time, that only lasted while we were actually in school or on the odd occasion, when we were walking home or on the train or something. Nearly every kid in this country now has their own mobile phone and as a consequence, the school bullies can hound them for as often as they like, even when they are in the 'safety' of their own bedrooms. You could just say, "Don't have a mobile phone in the first place," but let's be honest, they have become such an integral part of society that it would almost be like depriving that child of their liberty and they would become an outcast amongst their friends and fellow pupils. Can you imagine yourself all of a sudden without your own phone and access to the internet? On the odd occasions I've forgotten to take my mobile with me, it's almost like having my arm cut off and I feel

BIPOLAR…..MAYBE?
(Volume Two)

completely helpless. If you would have told me when I was a kid, that I could look up anything or watch or listen to anything from a small device that fits in my pocket, I would have said you were mad and living in a dream world, but that's exactly what's happened and we now depend on this technology so much, we can no longer remember what it was like to live without it.

It makes you wonder if kids actually read books anymore, rather than texts or snippets of information found on social media sites, because everything has to be so quick nowadays and sitting down with a good book requires at least a modicum of patience.

There was a really good television series on Channel 4 in the eighties called 'To the End of the Rhine' based on the book (or was it the other way round?) by the journalist Bernard Levin, which was also presented by him, and he discussed the art, history, food and architecture of the countries the river flows through. In one of the programmes, Levin visits a majestic looking library (sorry, I can't remember where it was or what it was called) and while browsing through some of the thousands and thousands of books, he discusses the advent of personal computers, which had just began appearing in the homes of a privileged few. He said that he could envisage a time when physical books didn't exist anymore, except perhaps in museums, and people would read straight from a computer screen rather than from a page. Little did he know how accurate his prediction would turn out to be, but instead of computer screens, books can now be read from a Kindle, with the text remarkably similar to that on a printed page.

"That will never happen," I told myself, "people will

always want to read paper books," and thankfully, that is still the case, even though Kindles are becoming more and more popular.

A day doesn't go by without my mum reading a book and she too dismissed the idea of a Kindle at first, that is until someone bought her one for a birthday present and now, she would never be without it. I can always remember when she first got the hang of using the Kindle and I went into the living room to give her a cup of tea. As I started to leave the room, I turned round to say something and saw her lick the tip of her finger before swiping along to the next page, as if she still had a physical book in her hand... bless her!

I have no problem with a Kindle and the fact you can read any book ever written, anywhere in the world, at any time and at the touch of a button, is absolutely amazing. I only hope physical books continue to be made and read and the billions of them lying in libraries are looked after and never lost.

Unfortunately, I don't get to read many books myself, I'm too busy writing them so I can bestow upon you my words of wisdom, but I bet if old Bernie Levin read one of my efforts, he would soon change his mind about cherishing them and they'd go straight into the bleedin' furnace.

I love watching those old sci-fi films from the 40's and 50's and whereas some of their predictions are correct, such as man (and woman) venturing into space or landing on the moon, most of the technology that is available to us nowadays, didn't even begin to enter their minds... I mean, how could it have? It was with the advent of the internet that things really began to

BIPOLAR…..MAYBE?
(Volume Two)

change and I wonder if computer scientist Tim Berners-Lee, who invented the World Wide Web, envisioned just how far and how quickly things would go and that people would be able to access everything on their mobile phones. It's funny, we still call them phones but the actual telephone part of the device is probably the least used, with people preferring to send texts rather than talk (for which I am guilty also)

I think that touchscreen devices have really made a positive contribution to technology as well and the idea of pressing buttons in this day and age, almost feels too basic and old fashioned to be taken seriously, and when we do now have to press a button, it's simulated on the screen rather than being a physical thing.

So, we now have smart phones, smart TV's, smart speakers, smart toilet paper (it won't be long, I tell you) and although all of those things are great (especially the toilet paper) I don't much like the idea of someone knowing exactly where you are when you are using them. For instance, you might be watching a programme on your smart TV and when the adverts come on and try to sell you something, like an even smarter TV or a cleverer mobile phone, the stores you can go to and purchase these things are specifically directed at you the viewer and they will be in a location close to where you live.

I was listening to the radio at work today (an ordinary radio with the only thing smart about it being that it tells you the time) and the DJ said you can tell your smart speaker to play Heart FM for you. Now I get the fact smart speakers are good for listening to any song you want, but to ask it to tune into a radio station is just plain lazy... all you have to do is press a button (yes, a real button... shock, horror!) or twiddle your knob (ooh er, missus!)

I can't understand why 'Tomorrow's World' isn't still shown on the telly anymore, because the things that are happening nowadays would make the programme more relevant than ever before and the presenters weren't too full of themselves either.

The whole thing is incredible and the technology of today could have come straight out of one of those old sci-fi films from the 40's or 50's... and round and round we go like a satellite circling the earth, like one of those old sci-fi films from the...

CHAPTER 38

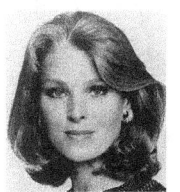

I was on a plane a few years back and sat behind two women who didn't stop talking for the whole duration of the two-and-a-half-hour flight. They seemed to be rabbiting on about members of their families and although I had no interest whatsoever in what they were saying, I couldn't help but overhear because they were talking so bleedin' loud.

"I thinking David is looking well," said the first woman.

"Yes," replied the other one, "he seems to have taken to fatherhood naturally"

"The kids are lovely I must admit, and well behaved too"

"I just wish his other half would cheer up a bit… I mean, she's got nothing to be miserable about"

"That's just her way and it comes across like that. Victoria is a nice person really because if she wasn't, he wouldn't put up with her"

"Either that or she wears the trousers in the relationship"

By this stage, I was losing the will to live and so decided to go to the toilet just to get a moment's peace and have a rest from hearing about their relatives. Standing up in the aisle, I walked past the two lady's seats and glanced down at them briefly, just to see what they looked like. It was then that I noticed one of those 'Hello' magazines or whatever crap these people look at, open on one of the women's laps, with a picture of David and Victoria Beckham plastered across the pages. I couldn't believe it because the two women had been talking like they knew the Beckham's personally and seemed to know every aspect of their lives and who said what to whom and all that rubbish.

After my breather in the toilet, I walked back to my seat and glancing down again, I saw a picture of Katie Price and her latest fella and knew I was in for a barrage of mindless gossip and wished I'd brought my iPod with me. It's bad enough having to hear about Katie Price but the TV is full of her antics as well and the only place I seem to be able to avoid that crap is by watching Al Jazeera. It's by far the best news channel out there and gives a balanced view on world events, unlike the BBC which now seems to spend much of its time plugging one of their TV shows like Strictly Come Dancing. I can honestly say that I've haven't watched a whole episode of Eastenders or Emmerdale or any of those other soaps and have never seen the X Factor or Britain's Got Talent or The Voice, Bake Off, Dance Off, Skate Off and Fuck Off! I admit I might have seen five minutes here and there if someone else is watching them in their own home, but even that's more than enough and I find myself having to leave the room.

It's not so much the contestants taking part in these programmes because many of them are clearly talented, it's the judges and presenters who love the sound of

BIPOLAR…..MAYBE?
(Volume Two)

their own voices and think they are so fucking self-righteous. Then you get programmes about people who don't clean their houses… I mean, who wants to stare at the TV and look at people living in pig styes or shows with such imaginative titles as 'My 200 Stone Wife' or 'Naked Ping Pong' or whatever?

Sorry, you must all think I'm a right old misery guts but I'm just not prepared to waste my life watching something I have absolutely no interest in, but I'm definitely not saying all TV programmes are bad. Yesterday is a good channel and I like shows about restoring cars and stuff, just as long as the presenter doesn't make the programme about him or herself. When Grand Designs first came on the air, I loved watching that but just like any popular programme, after a few years, more and more TV shows had the same idea, but I still think that's the best of the lot because Kevin McCloud really knows what he's talking about.

I'm able to get Netflix on my TV but apart from a few documentaries and some foreign films, by far the majority of it is absolute rubbish and there is no way I would ever subscribe to it (that's my sister's department)

If there is a film I really want to see (don't ask me how but I know if I'm going to like it or not before even seeing it) then I'll buy it on DVD or Blu-ray because when I do enjoy something, then I'll happily watch it more than once and you usually get some good extra features with them too. There are only a handful of film critics I'll pay attention to and thought Barry Norman was one of the best, when he hosted the 'Film' series

PART FOUR: WOULD THAT IT WERE

for many years. He was a proper critic, unlike those who followed him and why should I waste my time listening to people such as Claudia Winklepickers or whatever her bleedin' name is? Those types of presenters are film fans (much like myself) and being a fan of a film doesn't automatically make you a film critic.

I would begrudge paying for one of those streaming services, purely because I would have no interest in most of their content and until the day comes when you can stream absolutely any film or TV show, I'll stick to buying them. I honestly believe that the viewing standards of today are well below what they used to be and I love watching old BBC dramas (when they were good) from the seventies, eighties and early nineties. People have told me I should watch 'House of Cards' with Kevin Spacey and although I'm sure it's very good (he's a good actor) I'm a big fan of the original series with Ian Richardson (who was a brilliant actor) and I know I would be constantly comparing the American version to the British one, and finding faults with it. I always seem to end my books writing about films or TV shows (sorry about that) but I honestly think that if I had to sit through programmes I didn't like, they would slowly start to bring me down and that would mean months of feeling low, which is something I really don't want to happen. That's why I definitely don't want to be in a relationship ever again because I can do and watch whatever I want, whenever I want and if that means having a one-night stand here and there, then that's fine by me. Basically, after twenty years of marriage and bringing up the kids, I have slowly become increasingly selfish and it feels bloody good. I'm not putting pressure on someone to watch a film or TV show or listen to a song or album that's to my taste, and that person doesn't have to worry about me not enjoying their favourite things (lucky them!)

There's been me going on about having bipolar and how much I hate it (not so much in this book I grant you) when there are many, many people in the world who really do have terrible problems in their lives that make my own seem insignificant. It's always the poorer countries that seem to have natural disasters and famine or even wars due to their locations on the world map and when I sometimes wish I could win the lottery so I can at least buy a house, I think about those unfortunate people and realise just how lucky I am.

I've moaned about the things that make me feel miserable in life and that in turn can bring my mood down, whereas I should write about cheerful subjects just like Ian Dury did, because I haven't felt really happy in over six years and instead, have been in a kind of a limbo and not felt anything at all. Here goes…

Pinocchio walking in the sea, Fred Quimby and Tex Avery
Peter Paul Rubens and Austin Powers, Monty Python, Fawlty Towers
Señor Droopy, Jerry Mouse, banging music, especially House
Spike the dog and Tom the cat, James Cagney, "You dirty rat!"
Jimi Hendrix, Alvin Lee, a pint of lager, a Ford Capri

PART FOUR: WOULD THAT IT WERE

Betty Grable in 40's lockers, funny old men gone off their rockers
Odd One Out and Hide and Seek, Who Goes There? and Jesty week
Marty McFly, Doc Emmett Brown, Montgomery Burns, Krusty the Clown
Two reeler shorts, the best of Hal Roach, three Mini Coopers, Big William's coach
Cool Hand Luke's entire cast, memories of days gone past
Captain Beefheart, Country Joe, Eric Clapton, Let it Grow
Alfred Hitchcock, David Lean, Lindsey Buckingham, Peter Green
Buster Keaton, Harold Lloyd, the late Syd Barrett and Pink Floyd
Sean Connery as James Bond, a cute girl's arse, a leggy blonde
Stan and Ollie, James Finlayson, Richard Wright and Mr. Mason
A summers day, a gentle breeze, Setsuko Hara in Japanese
Paddington Bear with Michael Hordern, Buster Crabbe as Flash Gordon
Sergeant Bilko, Benny Hill, Ken Dodd live with time to kill
A shark called Bruce, his broken bite, Sherlock Holmes in black and white
Boris Karloff, a cup of Rosie, Lon Chaney Jr and Bela Lugosi
Country houses, castle moats, Fred C. Dobbs and Warren Oates

BIPOLAR…..MAYBE?
(Volume Two)

The Singing Detective and Pennies from Heaven, Akira Kurosawa, Samurai Seven

Clubber Lang is Mr. T, Jackie Wright, Henry McGee

Dr. Frankenstein, "It's alive!" Interstellar Overdrive

Spike Milligan said he was ill, Sidney Lumet on The Hill

A forgotten fiver found in my pocket, a 147 by The Rocket

Kate Reid in The Andromeda Strain, Margot Kidder, Lois Lane

An Ealing comedy with gentle humour, Fleetwood Mac starting a rumour

Lindsay Wagner, Jaime Sommers, mad Keith Moon and other drummers

Porridge Slade with Ronnie Barker, bad Count Dracula, Jonathan Harker

Humphrey Bogart, Lauren Bacall, Joe Don Baker, Walking Tall

Vinyl discs on metal tape, Einstein a Go-Go by Landscape

Janet Gaynor, Louise Brooks, Camilla Horn, their silent looks

Clocks go forward, blossom Springs, Nelson Riddle, Sinatra sings

A hedgehog's garden in the dark, the Mary Rose, the Cutty Sark

Desperate Dan and Minnie the Minx, John Schlesinger and his kitchen sinks

Alan Partridge, David Brent, cat paw prints in wet cement

Norbert Smith and Spinal Tap, Fred Dibnah with old cloth cap

PART FOUR: WOULD THAT IT WERE

The Rolling Stones, lips and licks, Tommy Cooper magic tricks
William Bendix, bouncing ball, Alan Ladd not too tall
Wayne and Radford feeling 'queer,' Robert Mitchum in Cape Fear
Glenda Jackson, Elizabeth R, Vanishing Point, Dodge Challenger car
Donald Fagen, colleague Walter, my two sons and my daughter
"Top of the world!" with Cody Jarrett, back at home with my ma Barrett.

I do actually feel a bit happier after that lot and should try doing it more often… shit, it's starting to wear off again!
So… what have you learned whilst perusing through the pages of this book…? I'll tell you, fuck all, that's what! It's just me going on about random things in my life which are probably meaningless to you, the poor reader who's had to sit through it, but don't worry 'cos there definitely won't be a 'Volume Three'

Oh god, I do miss the highs sometimes though, even if I complain about them. It would be great if I had a switch to turn my good moods on and off when I want, but I suppose that's asking too much and I just have to see what happens as each day passes.
I wanna go Yay and play and say… "La, La, La, La. Ding Dong, Ding Dong… BANG, BANG, BANG, BANG, BANG, BANG, BANG, BANG, BANG, BANG, BANG!" and say goodbye 'cos it's the end.
"Goodbye"

www.ingramcontent.com/pod-product-compliance
Lightning Source LLC
Chambersburg PA
CBHW071348210526
45465CB00001B/20